Allen's Fertility and Obstetrics in the Dog

LIBRARY OF VETERINARY PRACTICE

Editors
J.B. Sutton, JP, MRCVS
S.T. Swift, MA, VetMB, CertSAC

LIBRARY OF VETERINARY PRACTICE

Allen's Fertility and Obstetrics in the Dog

Second Edition

GARY C.W. ENGLAND
BVetMed, PhD, DVetMed, FRCVS, CertVA, DVR, DVReprod, DiplomateACT

Department of Farm Animal and Equine Medicine and Surgery
Royal Veterinary College
University of London
Hatfield, Herts
UK

Blackwell
Science

© 1992, 1998 by
Blackwell Science Ltd
Editorial Offices:
Osney Mead, Oxford OX2 0EL
25 John Street, London WC1N 2BL
23 Ainslie Place, Edinburgh EH3 6AJ
350 Main Street, Malden
  MA 02148 5018, USA
54 University Street, Carlton
  Victoria 3053, Australia

Other Editorial Offices:

Blackwell Wissenschafts-Verlag GmbH
Kurfürstendamm 57
10707 Berlin, Germany

Blackwell Science KK
MG Kodenmacho Building
7–10 Kodenmacho Nihombashi
Chuo-ku, Tokyo 104, Japan

First edition published 1992
Second edition published 1998

Set in 10/12pt Palatino
by DP Photosetting, Aylesbury, Bucks
Printed and bound in Great Britain by
MPG Books Ltd, Bodmin, Cornwall

DISTRIBUTORS

Marston Book Services Ltd
PO Box 269
Abingdon
Oxon OX14 4YN
(*Orders:* Tel: 01235 465500
        Fax: 01235 465555)

USA
Blackwell Science, Inc.
Commerce Place
350 Main Street
Malden, MA 02148 5018
(*Orders:* Tel: 800 759 6102
        781 388 8250
        Fax: 781 388 8255)

Canada
Copp Clark Professional
200 Adelaide Street West, 3rd Floor
Toronto, Ontario M5H 1W7
(*Orders:* Tel: 416 597 1616
        800 815 9417
        Fax: 416 597 1617)

Australia
Blackwell Science Pty Ltd
54 University Street
Carlton, Victoria 3053
(*Orders:* Tel: 03 9347 0300
        Fax: 03 9347 5001)

A catalogue record for this title
is available from the British Library

ISBN 0-632-04806-9

Contents

Preface

The first edition of this book was written by Dr W.E. Allen in the year before his death. Ed's aim was to produce a book that would be useful to veterinary students, and would be used in veterinary practice. The book was written with Ed's enthusiastic style and drew upon his large clinical experience and his brilliance as a teacher to produce a concise text that was practical and up-to-date.

As one of his former undergraduate and postgraduate students, I was delighted to be asked to revise the second edition of Ed's book and I hope that I have maintained the style and enthusiasm with which the first edition was written. During its preparation I have updated those sections in which new information has become available. The entire text has been revised and there are additional sections on the ultrasonographic examination of the reproductive tract, interpretation of hormone measurements, the fertilization period, the relation of semen quality to fertility, semen preservation and artificial insemination, and the pharmacological control of reproduction. I hope that this edition continues to be a useful source of practical information, but also that it stimulates further interest and debate in canine reproduction.

I am grateful to many people for their assistance in the revision of this book. However it is dedicated to my parents for giving 34 years of love, and is a tribute to the memory of Ed Allen, my teacher and friend.

Gary C.W. England

1 Anatomy of the Bitch's Reproductive Tract

greyhound - lg. clitoris due to testosterone admin. to impure rasing

1.1 VULVA *- ventral to the pelvic floor ; go dorsally when doing swabs, then horizontally*

- ❏ opening to female genital tract, bordered by the labia
- ❏ situated ventral to the floor of the pelvis
- ❏ derived embryologically from the urogenital sinus
- ❏ size depends on: (a) breed, (b) stage of oestrous cycle (Fig. 1.1)
- ❏ assessment of vulval size and tone can be useful for determining the fertile period

Size : estrogen → edema, puffed up

in heat - hard to see due to horizontal folds covering vulvar lips, esp in Eng. Bulldogs

1.2 VESTIBULE

ie posterior vagina

- ❏ potential tube which connects vulval opening to vagina
- ❏ on the ventral wall, cranial to the ventral vulval commissure, is the *clitoris* suspended in a transverse fold of mucosa
- ❏ the vestibular lumen runs cranially upwards 60° from the horizontal, and then a short distance forward in the pelvis to its junction with the vagina

1.3 VESTIBULO-VAGINAL JUNCTION

- ❏ in maiden bitches there is a constriction which indicates the position of the hymenal vestige
- ❏ in some bitches the hymen is totally or partially intact, thus preventing mating (see 14.3)
- ❏ the urethra opens just caudal to this region on the ventral floor

1.4 VAGINA

- ❏ directed cranially from the vestibulo-vaginal junction to the cervix (level with 4th or 5th lumbar vertebra) (Fig. 1.2)
- ❏ a potential tube lined by a stratified epithelium
- ❏ cranially this potential tube becomes narrow due to a dorsal median longitudinal fold of mucosa; the caudal end of this fold is often mistaken for the cervix (see 4.5)
- ❏ about 0.5–1.5 cm caudal to the cranial limit of the vagina, on its dorsal surface, is the os of the cervix

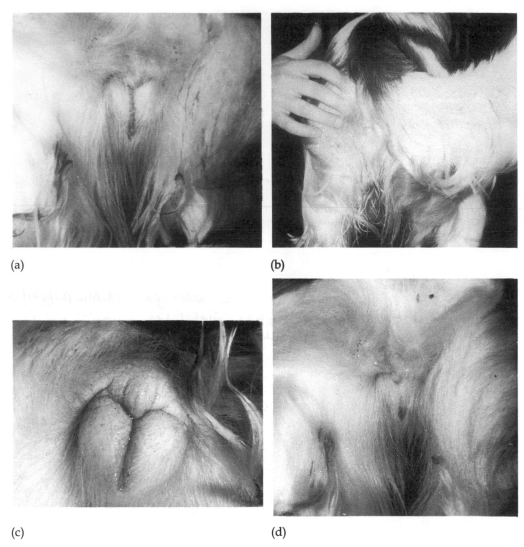

(a)   (b)

(c)   (d)

Fig. 1.1 Vulval changes during the oestrous cycle: (a) pro-oestrus, note the sero-sanguinous discharge at the vulva and on the hairs of the back leg; (b) oestrus, the tail is held to one side in response to pressure applied to the back or perivulval area; (c) oestrus, the vulva is swollen and discharge is still present; (d) early metoestrus, swelling is reduced but in this bitch the haemorrhagic discharge has persisted – this is not abnormal.

❏ the cranial two-thirds of the vagina is derived embryologically from the paired Müllerian ducts
❏ characteristics of the epithelium change in relation to the endocrine environment
❏ hypertrophy of the vaginal wall occurs during oestrus
❏ assessment of the degree of vaginal wall hypertrophy and epithelial proliferation can be useful for determining the fertile period

(a)

(b)   (c)

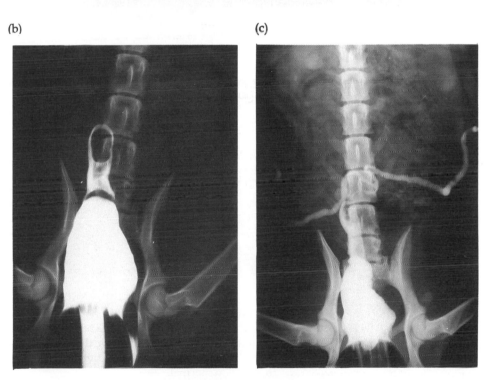

Fig. 1.2 Contrast radiography of the vagina and uterus: (a) lateral view of the vagina filled with contrast medium in a bitch in anoestrus, the cranial portion of the vagina (C) is narrower than the caudal part and the arrow points to the area where the cervix joins the vagina; (b) ventro-dorsal view of the vagina of the bitch in (a), note the length of the vagina. Distally there is incomplete filling of the vagina due to the cuff of a Foley catheter; (c) ventro-dorsal view of the vagina and uterus filled with contrast medium in a bitch in oestrus. (Reproduced by kind permission from the editor of the *Journal of Small Animal Practice*.)

, extremely soft & prone to damage

1.5   CERVIX UTERI

it is possible to cannulate the cervix

- ❏ a short, thick-walled organ with a narrow lumen which connects the vagina to the uterus
- ❏ the vaginal opening (os) opens dorsally into the cranial vagina
- ❏ ventral to the cervix is a blind-ending pouch of vagina
- ❏ the cervix enlarges during oestrus and can often be palpated trans-abdominally
- ❏ the cervical canal is patent during late pro-oestrus, oestrus, parturition and the post-partum period; at other times it is usually closed

1.6   UTERUS (Fig. 1.3)

- ❏ this is Y-shaped and composed of a short body (corpus) and two long horns (cornua)
- ❏ the body is connected to the cervix caudally and the tips of the horns communicate with the uterine (Fallopian) tubes cranially
- ❏ the length and width of the uterus is affected by both physiological and pathological (see 14.5) changes
- ❏ the uterine horns lengthen and begin to form folds during oestrus
- ❏ normal changes in the non-pregnant uterus are governed by circulating hormones, principally oestrogen and progesterone (see Chapter 3)

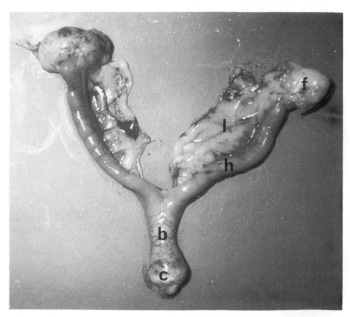

Fig. 1.3   Uterus and ovaries from a bitch in early pro-oestrus showing uterine horns (h), body (b) and cervix (c). The broad ligaments (l) are continuous with the mesovarium which contains (f) and surrounds the ovary.

Prepuberty

- ❏ the uterus is small in diameter
- ❏ uterine lumen is cross-shaped in section and the endometrial glands are simple and poorly developed
- ❏ the uterine vessels are small in size

Pro-oestrus

- ❏ the uterine vessels increase in size
- ❏ the endometrium becomes thicker and more oedematous
- ❏ the endometrial glands become more tortuous
- ❏ extravasation of erythrocytes occurs into the lumen of the uterus, the sero-sanguinous discharge passes via the cervix into the vagina

Oestrus

- ❏ the uterine vessels reach maximum size
- ❏ there is less endometrial oedema
- ❏ uterine glands become more numerous and tortuous
- ❏ extravasation of erythrocytes continues

Metoestrus (dioestrus)

- ❏ grossly the uterus has a 'twisted' (corkscrew) appearance associated with glandular proliferation but reduced oedema
- ❏ glandular proliferation continues until about the 30th day after ovulation
- ❏ in late metoestrus the glandular layer becomes more simple but often contains cystic dilations; the uterus is no longer twisted; leucocytes appear in the mucosa and necrotic epithelial tissue is seen in the lumen

Anoestrus

- ❏ the uterus has a similar appearance to prepuberty but is not as small in diameter

1.7 UTERINE (FALLOPIAN) TUBES

- ❏ run from the tip of the uterine horn to the ovary within the mesosalpinx and ovarian bursa
- ❏ composed of a narrow isthmus at the uterine end and a wider ampulla (where fertilization occurs) at the ovarian end
- ❏ terminate in fimbriae which are attached to the openings of the ovarian bursae – the fimbriae channel the ovulated ova into the uterine tube

1.8 OVARIES (Fig. 1.4)

- ❏ ovoid in shape when inactive and attached to the inner surface of the ovarian bursa

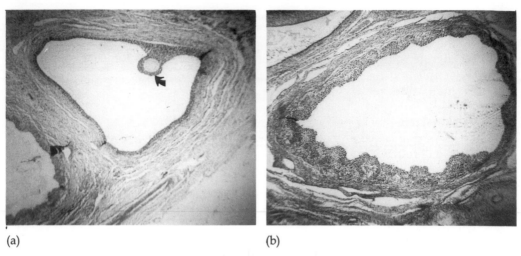

(a)   (b)

Fig. 1.4   Histology of the ovary: (a) a follicle in pro-oestrus containing an ovum (arrowed), the granulosa cell layer surrounding the follicle is relatively thin; (b) a follicle in early oestrus, the wall has luteinized and is producing progesterone but as yet this follicle has not ovulated.

❑ covered by a germinal epithelium, so that ovulation may occur anywhere on the surface of the ovary
❑ size depends on stage of the oestrous cycle

Prepuberty

❑ peripherally there is a layer of primordial follicles
❑ follicles may contain more than one ovum, although this is rare

Pro-oestrus

❑ follicles enlarge due to increasing size of their fluid-filled antra
❑ the granulosa is thrown into distinct folds
❑ plasma oestrogen concentrations increase from late anoestrus throughout pro-oestrus

Oestrus

❑ granulosa cells luteinize before ovulation
❑ this luteal tissue produces progesterone before ovulation
❑ ovulation usually occurs in early oestrus
❑ ova are released from follicles which do not collapse
❑ luteal tissue continues to proliferate

Metoestrus (dioestrus)

❑ the early corpus luteum is centrally cavitated
❑ progressive luteinization occurs from the wall inwards

❏ by about 20 days after ovulation the cavity of the corpus luteum is completely replaced by luteal cells

❏ after this time the corpora lutea gradually become smaller and the ovary is nodular in outline

Anoestrus

❏ remnants of corpora lutea remain for several months

❏ the significance of these luteal remnants is as yet uncertain

❏ small follicles are also present

❏ ovaries are bigger than before puberty but generally are small in size and have a flat surface

1.9 MESENTERY

❏ attaches the reproductive tract to the body wall, mainly dorsally

❏ the terminology of the various parts of this system is governed by their position and anatomical modifications:

Suspensory ligament: runs cranially from the ovary to the dorsal abdominal wall, level with the last rib; it is a strong fibrous structure

Mesovarium: bounded by the suspensory ligament cranially and continuous with the mesometrium caudally; composed of loose connective tissue containing fat and the ovarian vessels ·

Ovarian bursa: a pouch of the mesovarium which completely covers the ovary except for a small opening to the abdominal cavity; the fimbriae of the Fallopian tube are attached to this opening

Mesosalpinx: a fold of mesentery running between ovary and uterus, containing the uterine tube

Proper ligament of the ovary: a band of fibrous tissue which runs between the ovary and tip of the uterine horn, parallel to the mesosalpinx

Mesometrium: continuous with the mesovarium cranially; loose connective tissue containing the uterine vessels

1.10 BLOOD SUPPLY

❏ only the vessels encountered in routine surgical procedures are described

Ovarian artery and vein: arise from aorta and empty into the vena cava dorsal to the ovary (on the left the vein empties into the left renal vein); they do not communicate with uterine vessels

Uterine artery and vein: arise from the pudendal vessels near the vagina; they run cranially, parallel to each uterine horn to which they send regular branches

1.11 MAMMARY GLAND

- ❑ the number of mammary glands is variable
- ❑ glands are designated according to location: thoracic, abdominal, inguinal
- ❑ each gland has between 7 and 14 teat orifices
- ❑ mammary glands are small during anoestrus, pro-oestrus and oestrus
- ❑ approximately 35 days after ovulation there is obvious mammary gland development
- ❑ this development occurs in all bitches, even those without clinical signs of false pregnancy
- ❑ at this time milk production is common

bred ♀ c̄ @ least 6 mammary complexes
- each gland has 7-14 teat orifices
- MG enlarge in preg & nonpreg bitch at the end of the luteal phase
- always MG during routine physical

2 Physiology of the Oestrous Cycle

1st heat may be split & atypical in length or amt of vag-bleeding
- anywhere btwn 6 & 24 mos of age
- most fertile in 2nd part of heat

2.1 TERMINOLOGY

- ❑ this is confused in the bitch due to historical mistakes
- ❑ some terms are more acceptable because of traditional usage rather than scientific accuracy

2.2 PREPUBERTY

- ❑ the period between birth and the beginning of the first pro-oestrus
- ❑ can last from 6 to 24 months or more

2.3 PRO-OESTRUS *3-21d, avg 9d*

- ❑ lasts on average for 9 days but is very variable
- ❑ initial signs are swelling of the vulval lips and the appearance of a sero-sanguinous discharge from the vulva
- ❑ the quantity of discharge varies greatly and is of no clinical significance
- ❑ the discharge may not be seen in some bitches as they remove it by licking
- ❑ urination becomes more frequent (small quantities) to disseminate phero-mones produced by the vestibular mucosa
- ❑ the bitch is attractive to male dogs but will not usually allow coitus
- ❑ ovulation may occur towards the end of this period but normally occurs during oestrus

- attracted to males but doesn't allow mating

2.4 OESTRUS *range of 3-21 days*

bitches usually bred 11d or 13d.

- ❑ lasts on average 9 days but is very variable
- ❑ starts when bitch will first readily allow coitus
- ❑ ends when bitch refuses to allow coitus
- ❑ the discharge from the vulva may become less copious and less haemor-rhagic but this is not a constant feature, i.e. some bitches have scant dis-charge throughout pro-oestrus and oestrus, others have a copious 'bloody' discharge which persists after the end of oestrus
- ❑ ovulation usually occurs towards the beginning of oestrus; however, because behavioural responses are not consistent in bitches and the length of time that follicles take to develop is very variable, the following may happen:
  (a) ovulation may occur during a normal length pro-oestrus (as early as 7 days after the beginning)

1st drop of blood → out of heat
ovulation : 2-3 days after LH peak
cytology : 7 90% superficial cells

9

(b) ovulation may occur as early as 7 days after the onset of pro-oestrus and the bitch may be in oestrus at this time

(c) ovulation may occur as late as 30 days after the onset of pro-oestrus; the bitch is still receptive at this time

(d) ovulation may occur as late as 30 days after the onset of pro-oestrus; the bitch is not receptive at this time

❏ in addition, the time of ovulation may not be consistent during successive heats in the same bitch

❏ ovulations usually occur over a 72-hour period

❏ most ovulations occur 48–72 hours after the plasma peak of luteinizing hormone (see 3.3)

❏ because dog spermatozoa can live for up to 7 days in the bitch, and because ova are not ready for fertilization until 2–3 days after ovulation, bitches which are mated by more than one dog can have mixed litters

❏ in cases of paternity disputes genetic 'finger printing' is almost 100% accurate

2.5   METOESTRUS (DIOESTRUS) 55-60 days in length

79.01,
parabasal
cells

❏ the word metoestrus is traditionally used to describe the majority of the luteal phase of the bitch after the end of oestrus; there is little logical reason for this, and the word dioestrus is more accurate

❏ begins when the bitch first refuses coitus

-starts 1st
day of refusal

❏ lasts about 60 days and terminates when circulating progesterone concentrations become minimal (see 3.5); there is no clinical sign which heralds the end of metoestrus

❏ the vulva gradually becomes less swollen and any haemorrhagic discharge usually ceases during early metoestrus

❏ a mucoid vulval discharge may develop, as in pregnancy (see 11.5)

❏ pseudopregnancy (see 2.7) often occurs during late metoestrus

—ends o whelping or pseudopregnancy

2.6   ANOESTRUS

-ovarian
inactivity

-not part of
the cycle

❏ the period of ovarian inactivity between the end of metoestrus or pregnancy and the beginning of the next pro-oestrus

❏ can be very variable in length, i.e. from 1 month to 2 years, but is usually about 4 months

❏ length may be influenced by:

(a) time of year: some bitches retain the primitive tendency to one period of pro-oestrus/oestrus a year, e.g. the basenji; in other breeds more bitches may enter pro-oestrus/oestrus in spring than at other times

(b) pheromones: bitches kept together often exhibit pro-oestrus/oestrus around the same time; it is thought that odours from one oestrous bitch may stimulate others

(c) unknown factors: the signal responsible for causing follicular growth in most bitches is still a mystery

cyde <100 days =7hot enough time for uterus to repair = can r

2-11 mos - 1g breeds - long intervals

"Dormitory Effect" - ♀ tend to come into heat at

*25-30µg/kg (d) the advent of pro-oestrus may be predicted in so.
BD changes
for 1 week subQ ⟶ lutedyze =7 to kill C.L.

2.7 FALSE PREGNANCY (see also 17.8)
* NORMAL

❑ synonyms include phantom pregnancy, pseudopregnancy and pseudocyesis
❑ false pregnancy is common and normal
❑ caused by elevated plasma prolactin concentrations

*caused by ↑prolactin levels

❑ clinical signs include milk production and lactation, anorexia (but not weight loss), shivering, reluctance to leave the home, territorial aggression, nesting and mothering objects
❑ usually occurs 4-6 weeks after oestrus, but can occur at any time in some bitches

·no tx -can OHE

❑ represents a primitive mechanism for bitches to nurture other pups in the dog pack when pro-oestrus/oestrus occurs once a year, i.e. is synchronized
❑ usually regresses spontaneously in 10-30 days
❑ sometimes requires treatment if owners cannot cope with the clinical change in the bitch or if she develops mastitis
❑ there is usually only one episode of false pregnancy after each oestrus, but when hormone therapy is used, repeated bouts may occur (see 24.1)
❑ although normal, false pregnancy is also discussed under endocrinological abnormalities (see 17.8)

-also see inspays done during luteal phase

Some myths about false pregnancy

Progesterone

❑ it is still said by some that progesterone is the cause of false pregnancy; this is not true because:
(a) false pregnancy can be treated with progestogens (see 24.1)

'strogerol Testosterone:
-Danger of hormamon depression

(b) bitches with false pregnancy do not have higher circulating concentrations of progesterone than others at the same stage of the cycle
(c) bitches with false pregnancy do not produce progesterone for longer than others
(d) bitches with false pregnancy do have raised prolactin blood concentrations
(e) signs of false pregnancy can be suppressed by giving drugs that inhibit prolactin secretion (e.g. bromocriptine and cabergoline (see 24.1))

ndrogen:
tibolerone
(oral liq)
-safe, reduces objectional signs
-given at the end of luteal phase

Overt and covert false pregnancies

❑ it is often said that all bitches have a false pregnancy which in some is overt and in others is covert; this is not true and confusion has arisen due to the terminology used in other species
❑ all bitches have mammary swelling and the production of some milk
❑ the clinical signs of pseudopregnancy encompass a large range with some bitches showing no signs and others exhibiting marked behavioural changes

Prolactin inhibitors: Bromocriptine
-can do nothing to prevent false preg. unless you want to do an OHE

❏ most cases can be considered physiological and normal and it is often the concern of the owner that governs which animals require treatment

The situation in the cat and rat should not be confused with that in the dog:

❏ dogs are spontaneous ovulators (mating is not required)
❏ corpora lutea function for about 60–70 days in pregnant and non-pregnant bitches; in non-pregnant bitches this period of time is termed metoestrus or dioestrus (see 2.5)
❏ it is incorrect to refer to the luteal phase *per se* of the bitch as a false pregnancy
❏ clinical signs of false pregnancy do occur in some bitches during metoestrus; they are not directly related to progesterone concentrations in the blood

Pyometra

❏ it is sometimes said that bitches that have false pregnancies are more prone to pyometra; this is not true but:
(a) false pregnancy and pyometra occur at the same stage of the cycle (metoestrus)
(b) a bitch that has had progestogen treatments for false pregnancies may be more likely to develop pyometra as a result

Irregular oestrous cycles

❏ it is sometimes said that bitches with irregular oestrous cycles are more likely to develop false pregnancies; this is not true

Litter

❏ it is sometimes said that allowing a bitch to have a litter will stop subsequent false pregnancies; this is not true

Ovariohysterectomy

❏ it is sometimes thought that bitches which have signs of false pregnancy after ovariohysterectomy have ovarian tissue which has not been removed; this may be true but:
(a) most false pregnancies that occur after ovariohysterectomy are the result of surgery just before or during a false pregnancy. Removal of the ovaries causes plasma progesterone concentration to decline and results in a surge release of prolactin
(b) if a bitch does have a false pregnancy after ovariohysterectomy it may be preceded by a period of oestrus if ovarian tissue is present

Pseudopregnancy –
Tx – synthetic progesterone
testosterone

Hypothalamus
↓ GnRH (pulsatile manner)
Pituitary
FSH ↓   ↓ LH - maturation
follicle growth   luteinization
                              ovulation of
                              follicles

3 Endocrinology of the Oestrous Cycle

3.1 GONADOTROPHIN-RELEASING HORMONE (GnRH, LHRH)

- released in a pulsatile manner in the hypothalamus
- reaches the anterior pituitary gland via a specialized (portal) blood circulation
- attaches to the cells which produce follicle-stimulating hormone (FSH) (see 3.2) and luteinizing hormone (LH) (see 3.3) to stimulate their production and release; it is thought that differences in pulse quality select for FSH or LH release
- the effect on the receptors is transient because binding affinity is low; GnRH is rapidly released by the receptors and quickly metabolized
- synthetic analogues or agonists of GnRH have been developed; these have increased potency due to their ability to remain attached to binding sites and to resist metabolism; after initial stimulation, agonists cause inactivity of gonadotrophin-producing cells because pulsatile stimuli are prevented
- other analogues of GnRH, the antagonists, have been developed to compete for binding sites and block endogenous activity; these are expensive and may not cause initial stimulation

3.2 FOLLICLE-STIMULATING HORMONE (FSH)

- a gonadotrophin produced by and released from the anterior pituitary gland
- it is responsible for the stimulation of the growth of follicles in the ovaries
- factors which initiate its release are not known
- circulating concentrations in bitches are not well documented

3.3 LUTEINIZING HORMONE (LH)

— luteotrophic - maintains the fxn of corpora lutea
LH output is very short lived → hard to determine that it has happened

- a gonadotrophin produced in and released from the pituitary gland
- it is released in short bursts or pulses
- increased pulse frequencies occur 1–2 weeks before the beginning of pro-oestrus
- stimulates the maturation, luteinization and ovulation of ovarian follicles
- circulating concentrations rise rapidly to reach a peak about 48 hours before the majority of ovulations (ovulations may occur over a 72-hour period)
- this peak occurs usually in late pro-oestrus or early oestrus (Fig. 3.1) (see 2.4)
- this hormone is also luteotrophic (maintains the function of corpora lutea)

— LH levels ↑ rapidly to reach a peak ~48 hrs.
before the majority of ovulations
— peak usually occurs in late proestrus or early estrus

13

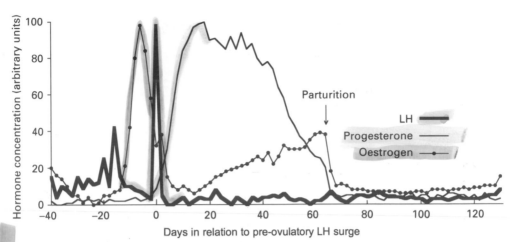

Fig. 3.1   Schematic representation of the main hormonal events during the pregnant oestrous cycle.

[handwritten margin note: + endo]

3.4   OESTROGENS *- peak just before LH peaks*

- ❑ steroid hormones produced in the bitch by growing follicles
- ❑ mainly 17α-oestradiol, 17β-oestradiol and oestrone, some of which may be conjugated
- ❑ circulating concentrations rise a little for a few days before the beginning of pro-oestrus
- ❑ a sharp rise in blood concentrations occurs later, resulting in a peak about 48 hours before the surge of LH (Fig. 3.1)
- ❑ oestrogens cause the changes which occur in pro-oestrus, (see 2.3):
  - (a) vaginal discharge (uterine bleeding)
  - (b) thickening of the vaginal mucosa
  - (c) change in cervical mucus consistency
  - (d) vulval swelling
  - (e) pheromone production
  - (f) behavioural changes

*[handwritten margin note: *only useful hormone for timing breeding]*

3.5   PROGESTERONE *- goes up to ~2 ng around the LH peak / ↑ occurs extremely rapidly*

- ❑ a steroid hormone produced by mature follicles and corpora lutea
- ❑ circulating concentrations start to rise around the time of the oestrogen peak (Fig. 3.1); the hormone is produced by luteinizing granulosa cells in the unruptured follicles (this is unusual compared with many domestic mammals)
- ❑ plasma values increase steadily and are significantly raised by the time of ovulation (see 2.4)
- ❑ maximal concentrations are reached about 20 days after the end of oestrus, whether the bitch is pregnant or not

[handwritten margin note: ~60-70 days' sharp ↓ of progesterone → triggers prolactin]

[handwritten: dog ovulate a diploid ovum → must expel a polar body before it is fertilized.]

[handwritten: penetration → fusion & fertilization occurs later]

- ❑ a gradual decline in values then occurs until they become basal at about 60–70 days after ovulation
- ❑ the luteal phase is almost identical in pregnancy and non-pregnancy; in fact the non-pregnant luteal phase is slightly longer and progesterone concentrations are slightly lower than in pregnancy (Fig. 3.2)

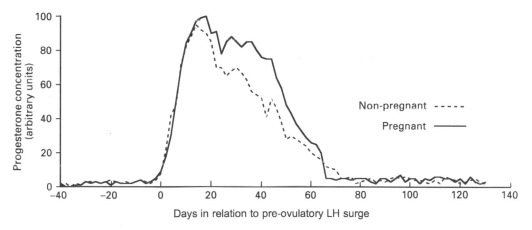

Fig. 3.2 Schematic representation of the plasma progesterone profile during pregnancy and non-pregnancy.

3.6 PROLACTIN

- ❑ produced in and released by the anterior pituitary gland
- ❑ it acts on the mammary gland (primed by the actions of oestrogens and progesterone) to stimulate milk production
- ❑ blood concentrations usually rise as concentrations of progesterone fall, although in some instances progesterone can stimulate prolactin release
- ❑ prolactin causes signs of pseudo-pregnancy (see 2.7 and 24.1, 24.8)
- ❑ in nursing bitches, blood concentrations of prolactin are very high for some time after parturition
- ❑ prolactin is also luteotrophic (maintains the function of corpora lutea)

3.7 ANDROGENS

- ❑ the functions of these hormones in the bitch are unknown
- ❑ testosterone concentrations in the blood peak at the same time as LH during oestrus
- ❑ androstenedione concentrations are high during metoestrus and pregnancy, and closely follow those of progesterone

3.8 PROSTAGLANDINS *[handwritten: kills CL]*

- ❑ spontaneous prostaglandin production by the uterus is not responsible for causing lysis of the corpora lutea at the end of the non-pregnant luteal phase, as in other species

❏   in the non-pregnant bitch corpora lutea appear to become non-functional gradually, due either to lack of trophic support (possibly LH and/or prolactin) or because they have an inherent lifespan

❏   in the pregnant bitch, however, prostaglandin causes final lysis of the corpora lutea and the initiation of parturition. At this time the corpora lutea are producing very little progesterone compared with earlier in pregnancy

Prostaglandin - kills CL
              - labor
              - opens cervix

- cycle of the bitch is
  not controlled by PG
  as in other species
- very little PGF
  produced by
  uterus, only use is in
  preg ♀.

- injecting GnRH → no response

4 Clinical Examination of the Bitch's Reproductive Tract

4.1 BASIC EXAMINATION OF THE REPRODUCTIVE TRACT

This consists of:

- ❏ visual examination of the perineum and vulva
- ❏ palpation of the mammary glands
- ❏ collection of vaginal cells for the study of vaginal exfoliative cytology
- ❏ digital examination of the vestibule and caudal vagina
- ❏ endoscopic examination of the vestibule, vagina and cervix
- ❏ real-time ultrasonographic imaging
- ❏ measurement of plasma hormone concentrations

4.2 ADDITIONAL TECHNIQUES THAT MAY BE CONSIDERED

These include:

- ❏ bacteriological examination of the reproductive tract *Vg. culture*
- ❏ endocrinological stimulation tests
- ❏ laparoscopy or laparotomy techniques
- ❏ karyotyping

4.3 VISUAL EXAMINATION OF THE PERINEUM

- ❏ may allow the stage of the oestrous cycle to be predicted (see Fig. 1.1)
- ❏ may allow the detection of intersexual abnormalities (see Chapter 16)

4.4 PALPATION OF THE MAMMARY GLANDS

- ❏ mammary glands are usually small during anoestrus and pro-oestrus
- ❏ mammary gland size may be large in multiparous bitches
- ❏ approximately 35 days after ovulation there is increased size of the mammary glands:
  - (a) at this time there is often milk production
  - (b) pseudopregnancy is common and normal

4.5   VAGINAL CYTOLOGY

Histological changes in the vaginal epithelium

Prepuberty and anoestrus

❑ consists of two layers, the outer of which appears pseudostratified
❑ there is no leucocytic infiltration

Pro-oestrus

❑ gradually becomes a stratfied squamous, epithelium
❑ about 16 cells thick at the end of pro-oestrus
❑ hyperplasia, hypertrophy and mitoses are seen in the basal layers
❑ the superficial squamous cells become keratinized
❑ there is no leucocytic infiltration

Oestrus

❑ the stratified squamous epithelium gradually sloughs
❑ there is no leucocytic infiltration

Metoestrus (dioestrus)

❑ thickness is 3–6 cells
❑ the epithelium and lamina propria are infiltrated with polymorphonuclear leucocytes
❑ by mid metoestrus the epithelium is two cells thick and cellular infiltration has subsided

Exfoliative cytology (Fig. 4.1)

❑ this term is incorrect because assessment is also made of bacterial and erythrocyte (uterine origin) numbers

Anoestrus

❑ *epithelial cells:* these are mainly round cells with active nuclei and a small cytoplasm. The smaller cells (parabasal cells) originate close to the basement membrane of the mucosa; the larger cells are produced by cell division and are known as intermediate cells
❑ *polymorphonuclear leucocytes:* usually present in small to moderate numbers
❑ *erythrocytes:* absent
❑ *bacteria:* usually absent

Pro-oestrus

❑ *epithelial cells:* immediately before, and also during, early pro-oestrus the number of large intermediate cells in the smear increases; towards the end of

pro-oestrus there is an increase in the proportion of cells which are becoming keratinized, i.e. more straight sided and with smaller nucleus
- *polymorphonuclear leucocytes:* present in small numbers initially but gradually decrease; usually absent at the end of pro-oestrus
- *erythrocytes:* usually very many throughout, but numbers of no clinical significance; sometimes they are lysed in smear preparation
- *bacteria:* numbers of bacteria (seen with some stains only) increase throughout pro-oestrus

Oestrus

- *epithelial cells:* early in oestrus maximal cornification (keratinization) occurs, i.e. between 60 and 90% of cells are straight sided and have small (pyknotic) nuclei or no nucleus (they are then called squames)
  NB: a 'false' peak of cornification sometimes occurs before the real peak; this can be recognized by the vague (pale staining) nature of the squames – the cause of this is unknown but it is not reported by those who use trichrome stains
- *polymorphonuclear leucocytes:* usually absent until the end of oestrus
- *erythrocytes:* may be absent, few or many; numbers are of no clinical significance
- *bacteria:* present usually in large numbers until the end of oestrus

Metoestrus (dioestrus)

- *epithelial cells:* at the end of oestrus all the epithelial cells are intermediate or parabasal, and are present in large numbers; as metoestrus proceeds cell numbers decrease and cells are similar to those in anoestrus
- *polymorphonuclear leucocytes:* at the end of oestrus there is a massive influx of these cells; as metoestrus proceeds, numbers decrease but some are always present
- *erythrocytes:* usually absent but may be seen in early metoestrus and are of no clinical significance
- bacteria: disappear dramatically at end of oestrus, coincident with influx of neutrophils and the appearance of mucus and debris
NB: vaginal smears are similar in metoestrus and pregnancy

Preparation of vaginal smears

Collection of vaginal material

Bacteriological swab

- insert a bacteriological swab into the vestibule and caudal vagina to absorb exudate; gently roll the swab onto a microscope slide
- this method is not ideal because:
  (a) vestibular cells are also collected

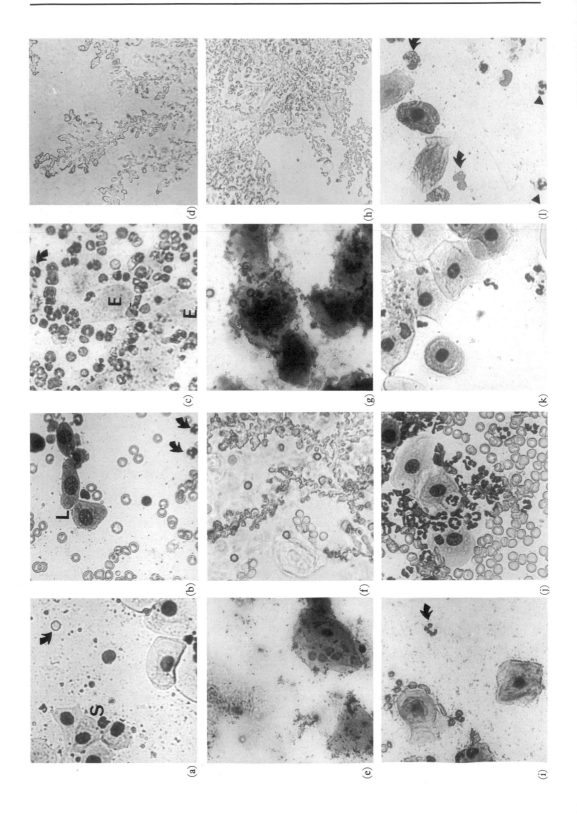

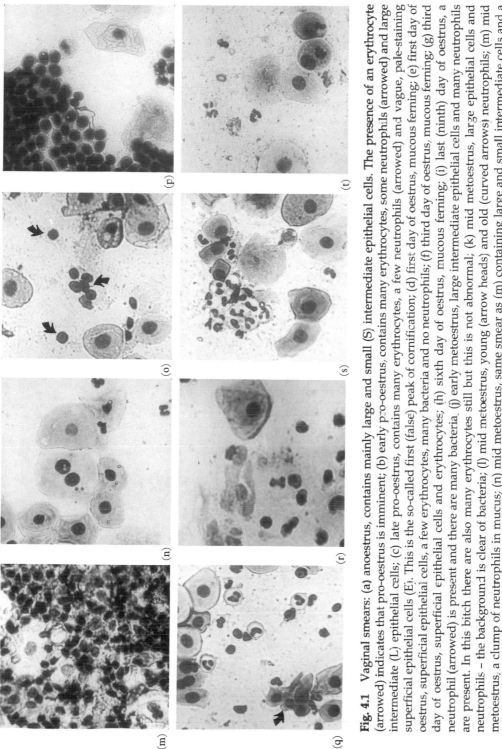

Fig. 4.1 Vaginal smears: (a) anoestrus, contains mainly large and small (S) intermediate epithelial cells. The presence of an erythrocyte (arrowed) indicates that pro-oestrus is imminent; (b) early pro-oestrus, contains many erythrocytes, some neutrophils and large intermediate (L) epithelial cells; (c) late pro-oestrus, contains many erythrocytes, a few neutrophils (arrowed) and vague, pale-staining superficial epithelial cells (E). This is the so-called first (false) peak of cornification; (d) first day of oestrus, mucous ferning; (e) first day of oestrus, superficial epithelial cells, a few erythrocytes, many bacteria and no neutrophils; (f) third day of oestrus, mucous ferning; (g) third day of oestrus, superficial epithelial cells and erythrocytes; (h) sixth day of oestrus, mucous ferning; (i) last (ninth) day of oestrus, a neutrophil (arrowed) is present and there are many bacteria. (j) early metoestrus, large intermediate epithelial cells and many neutrophils are present. In this bitch there are also many erythrocytes still but this is not abnormal; (k) mid metoestrus, large epithelial cells and neutrophils – the background is clear of bacteria; (l) mid metoestrus, young (arrow heads) and old (curved arrows) neutrophils; (m) mid metoestrus, a clump of neutrophils in mucus; (n) mid metoestrus, same smear as (m) containing large and small intermediate cells and a few neutrophils; (o) anoestrus, it is not known whether the round 'cells' (arrowed) are lymphocytes or the nuclei of epithelial cells; (p) anoestrus, the group of small epithelial cells (arrowed) resemble endometrial cells or sheets of endometrial cells; (q) anoestrus, the group of small epithelial cells may be parabasal vaginal epithelial cells or sheets of endometrial cells; (r) vaginitis, not all the cell types are seen in normal smears; (s) vaginitis, this bitch was attractive to male dogs, had a swollen vulva and was thought to be in oestrus; (t) pregnancy, this bitch was known to be pregnant but was attractive to male dogs and had a mucoid discharge.

(b) in metoestrus and anoestrus mucus is collected; this dries (fixes) slowly on the slide and causes distortion of cells

(c) the physical rolling of the swab on the slide causes cell disruption

(d) elements from the swab are included in the smear

❏ the method can be improved by using a speculum or cylindrical guide to prevent contamination with vestibular cells

Spatula

❏ scrape material from the vaginal wall using a metal spatula

❏ this method is not ideal because:

(a) very little material is collected

(b) the material is difficult to spread over the microscope slide

Aspiration

❏ aspirate material from the caudal vagina using a catheter or pipette; place a drop of exudate on a microscope slide and spread as a blood smear

❏ during metoestrus and anoestrus a small amount of saline can be introduced into the vagina and reaspirated, to collect a suspension of cells; if the smear is made and dried immediately, cell distortion does not occur

❏ this method produces a clear undistorted smear, and the collected material can also be used for examination of mucus crystallization in oestrus (see pp. 24–25, 74)

Staining vaginal smears

Shorr's method

❏ advantages:

(a) differentiates between keratinized (orange) and non-keratinized (blue) epithelial cells

(b) from this an index of keratinization (eosinophilic index) can be calculated

❏ disadvantages:

(a) there is no absolute value of the eosinophilic index which indicates ovulation time

(b) the staining method is complicated and very time consuming if individual stains are used, and components require regular filtering or renewal

NB: trichrome stains like Shorr's are excellent for human vaginal cytology where many slides are processed each day; bitch vaginal smears are usually taken too infrequently to justify the use of a complicated staining technique

Methylene blue

❏ pour the stain onto an air dried slide for 5–20 minutes; wash off excess stain with water and examine immediately

❏ advantages:

(a) very simple

(b) rapid
❏ disadvantages:
(a) must examine the wet slide inmediately, as drying causes distortion of the cells
(b) examining wet slides under high power may cause condensation on the objective lens
(c) no permanent record of the slides can be kept

Leishman's stain

❏ flood the air dried slide with 2 ml stain and leave for 2–3 minutes
❏ add 2 ml of phosphate buffer gently so that surface tension prevents dripping; a metallic sheen will be seen on the surface of the diluted stain
❏ after 20 minutes wash off stain with water and allow to dry
❏ advantages:
(a) relatively simple
(b) quick
❏ disadvantage: the slide will dry if forgotten

Diff-Quik (Merz and Dade)

❏ the slide (air dried) is dipped six times into each of three solutions, washed immediately with water and allowed to dry
❏ advantages:
(a) rapid
(b) gives consistent results
❏ disadvantages:
(a) expensive
(b) one solution (fixer) evaporates rapidly (even if not used)
(c) solutions must be changed frequently

Interpretation of vaginal smears

Determination of optimal mating time (see also Chapter 10)

❏ this is an indirect method of monitoring hormonal events (particularly oestrogen – see 3.4); the scope for anticipating future changes is limited
❏ vaginal cytology can only be useful for indicating the fertile period and not the fertilization period (see 10.2)
❏ take the first smear about 5 days after the first observed signs of pro-oestrus, as some bitches may be close to ovulation at this time (see 2.4)
❏ depending on the cellular content, repeat the smears every 2–3 days
❏ calculate the percentage of anuclear cells:

$$\text{anuclear cell index} = \frac{\text{no. anuclear cells}}{\text{total number epithelial cells}} \times 100$$

❏ mating should be recommended when usually more than 80% of cells are

anuclear and there is an absence of polymorphonuclear leucocytes (Fig. 10.2)
- ❏ the sudden decrease in the anuclear cell index, and a return of a large number of polymorphonuclear leucocytes denotes the end of the fertilization period

Diagnosis of vaginitis (see 14.3 and Fig. 4.1)

- ❏ excess vulval discharge suggests vaginal or uterine disease
- ❏ male dogs are often interested in bitches with vulval discharge, even when they are not in oestrus
- ❏ it is difficult to define vaginitis in the bitch because there are polymorphonuclear leucocytes present at all stages except during oestrus
- ❏ very large numbers of polymorphonuclear leucocytes in vaginal smears suggest uterine disease (pyometra: endometrial cells may also be seen)
- ❏ many vulval discharges are normal, i.e. during metoestrus and pregnancy, and may just indicate increased mucus production
- ❏ many bitches considered to have excessive vulval discharge have very few polymorphonuclear leucocytes in vaginal smears
- ❏ bacteriological findings are discussed later
- ❏ vaginal smears are invaluable for distinguishing bitches which are in pro-oestrus/oestrus from bitches which are otherwise attractive to male dogs

Pregnancy diagnosis

- ❏ vaginal smears can *not* be used as a method of pregnancy diagnosis
- ❏ smears will *not* distinguish between metoestrus, pregnancy and anoestrus

Crystallization (ferning) patterns in vaginal (cervical) mucus (Fig. 4.1)

Collection of samples

- ❏ vaginal secretion is best collected by pipette or catheter as described on p. 22
- ❏ place a drop of exudate on a slide and hold the slide vertically to allow the drop to 'run'
- ❏ do not examine until the slide is *completely* dry
- ❏ examine under × 40 objective with the condenser lowered

Interpretation of mucus crystallization

- ❏ the smear is examined for both the type of ferning pattern and the area of the smear covered by this pattern
- ❏ the ferning pattern is scored arbitrarily using five classes from minor ferning (with short stems and irregular stellate patterns) to bold ferning (with long stems and clear venation and subvenation)
- ❏ the surface area is scored using five classes from less than 1% cover, to greater than 20% cover
- ❏ the two scores may be added to calculate the ferning index (values 0–10)

[handwritten at top: opaque grey/bloody vag. discharge → neoplasia / stumppyometra / ovarian remnant syndrome]

- ferning is most intense and covers a greater area of the smear after the second peak of cornification of epithelial cells; it may therefore help differentiate the first and second peak
- individual bitches do not always reach a peak ferning index score of 10
- vaginal washings will give erroneous results due to the addition of water; with this method, crystallization can be seen in metoestrous samples

[handwritten: Visual exam of perineum - intersex? amt of vulvar swelling, amt + colour of discharge]

4.6 DIGITAL EXAMINATION OF THE REPRODUCTIVE TRACT

- clean the vulva and insert a lubricated gloved finger
- the vestibule is directed upwards to the vagina
- the external urethral orifice can be palpated ventrally
- vagina is dry in anoestrus and metoestrus (dioestrus), but moist during pro-oestrus and oestrus
- may detect hymenal remnants or abnormalities of the vestibulo-vaginal junction (strictures, see 14.3)
- may detect hyperplasia of the vaginal floor during oestrus (see 14.3)

[handwritten: - strictures difficult to diag. during dioestrus or early oestrus]

4.7 ENDOSCOPIC EXAMINATION OF THE FEMALE REPRODUCTIVE TRACT

[handwritten: - difficult unless in oestrus - use flexible endoscope - adequate vag. distension essential - may be used to time breeding.]

- bitches in oestrus may allow endoscopic examination with or without sedation; at other times general anaesthesia may be necessary
- auriscopes, even with long nozzles, are too short for thorough examination
- most bitch vaginal speculae also only reach to the vestibulo-vaginal junction
- rigid cold-light endoscopes and those with flexible fibreoptics give best results but:
  (a) it may be difficult to focus on the vaginal wall unless the canal is distended with air or water
  (b) the caudal limit of the dorsal median fold may be mistaken for the cervix
  (c) the cranial half of the vagina is very narrow, especially in the non-oestrous bitch, and may be difficult to visualize (see Fig. 1.2)
  (d) on many occasions the vaginal os of the cervix will not be seen
  (e) examination to elucidate the cause of abnormal discharge is usually unrewarding
- vaginal endoscopy may be useful for the assessment of the optimal mating time (see Chapter 10) and certain cases of reproductive tract disease

Interpretation

- *anoestrus:* vaginal folds are flat and may disappear when the vagina is insufflated; they appear red due to the underlying capillaries
- *pro-oestrus:* vaginal folds become larger, rounder, moister and paler; sanguineous discharge is seen between the folds
- *early oestrus:* the folds become wrinkled and subdivided into smaller rounder folds

❑ *late oestrus:* the secondary folds become angulated and the vagina appears dry

❑ *metoestrus:* the folds become rounded and less distinct and the mucosa appears patchy due to loss of the cornified layer

4.8 ULTRASONOGRAPHIC EXAMINATION OF THE FEMALE REPRODUCTIVE TRACT

Principles of diagnostic ultrasound

❑ diagnostic ultrasound utilizes sound frequencies between 2 and 10 MHz

❑ ultrasound is produced by application of an alternating voltage to piezo-electric crystals which change in size and produce a pressure or ultrasound wave. Returning echoes deform the same crystals which generate a surface voltage

❑ most diagnostic ultrasound machines use the principle of brightness modulation (B-mode) where the returning echoes are displayed as dots, the brightness of which is proportional to their amplitude

❑ real-time B-mode ultrasound is a dynamic imaging system where informatiuon is continually updated and displayed on a monitor

❑ ultrasound is attenuated within tissues and attenuation is related to wavelength of the sound, the density of the tissue, the heterogenicity of the tissue and the number and type of echo interfaces

❑ bright (specular) echoes are produced when a large proportion of the beam is reflected back to the transducer; these echoes are displayed as white areas on the ultrasound machine screen

❑ no echoes are produced when the sound is transmitted and not reflected; these areas are displayed as black on the ultrasound machine screen

❑ non-specular echoes are produced when the beam encounters a structure similar to one wavelength in size, and these echoes appear as varying shades of grey on the ultrasound machine screen

The ultrasound transducer

❑ piezoelectric crystals are arranged together to form an ultrasound transducer, contained within the ultrasound head

❑ the crystals may be arranged:
(a) in a line (linear array transducer)
(b) in an arc (sector transducer)
(c) in an arc and electronically triggered (phased array transducer)
(d) mounted upon a rotating wheel (mechanical sector transducer)

❑ transducers produce sound of a characteristic frequency:
(a) high frequencies allow good resolution although there is greater attenuation of the sound beam in tissues
(b) low frequencies allow a greater depth of penetration (less attenuation) but with reduced resolution

Equipment for examination of the bitch

❏ sector transducers are most suited to transabdominal imaging
❏ for the examination of the ovaries and of early pregnancy a 7.5 MHz transducer is most suitable
❏ for the examination of later pregnancy a 5.0 MHz transducer is necessary
❏ a 5.0 MHz transducer offers a compromise which gives a reasonable depth of penetration combined with adequate tissue resolution
❏ the ultrasound machine should have a keyboard to allow identification of the animal and possess electronic callipers to allow measurement of images
❏ there should be facilities to record the images and this can be achieved using:
   (a) a thermal printer
   (b) a Polaroid camera
   (c) a multiformat camera

Ultrasound terminology

❏ tissues that markedly reflect sound (such as gas, bone and metal) appear white on the ultrasound screen and are called echogenic
❏ tissues that transmit sound (such as fluid) appear black on the ultrasound screen and are called anechogenic (or anechoic)
❏ tissues that allow some transmission and some reflection (such as most soft tissues) appear as varying shades of grey and are called hypoechogenic or hyperechogenic depending upon their exact appearance
❏ strictly, a hyperechogenic tissue produces a hyperechoic region within the image, although these terms are often used synonymously

Examination of the bitch

❏ clipping the hair of the ventral abdomen is required for examination of the uterine body and horns
❏ clipping of the hair over the flank is often necessary to image the ovaries
❏ in many patients imaging is most conveniently performed with the bitch in the standing position

The normal non-pregnant uterus

❏ lies dorsal to the bladder, but its position may be variable depending upon:
   (a) the extent of bladder filling
   (b) the size of the uterus
   (c) the stage of the reproductive cycle
❏ the uterine body of the pre-pubertal and non-pregnant bitch during anoestrus may be less than 1 cm in transverse diameter
❏ the uterus may be identified dorsal or dorso-lateral to the bladder, and can be shown to be tubular by imaging in two perpendicular planes (Fig. 4.2)
❏ the uterus may be more readily imaged in older multiparous bitches
❏ in older bitches the bifurcation and distal uterine horns can be detected in approximately 40% of cases

difficult to visualize in young

edema during estrus not prominent as in horses

(a)

(b)

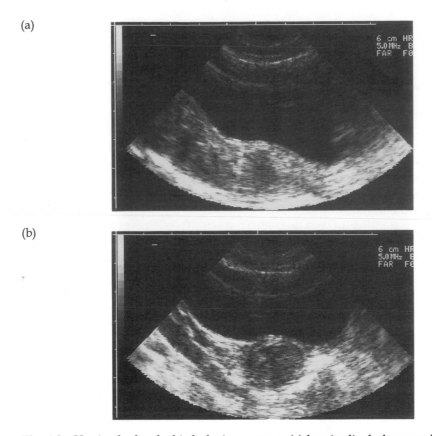

Fig. 4.2 Uterine body of a bitch during oestrus: (a) longitudinal ultrasound image, the uterus lies dorsal to the anechoic bladder (ventral in this image since the bitch was in the standing position with the transducer adjacent to the ventral abdominal wall), and has a rectangular appearance; (b) transverse ultrasound image, the uterus has a circular appearance and the hypo- and hyperechoic layers can be easily identified (5.0 MHz transducer, scale in centimetres).

❑ the uterine body and horns are composed of two distinct layers (Fig. 4.2):
   (a) a central homogeneous relatively hypoechoic region (endometrium)
   (b) a peripheral hyperechoic layer (serosa)
❑ during oestrus the uterus becomes increasingly hypoechoic and develops central radiating hyperechoic lines
❑ the changes in uterine echotexture are associated with an increase in uterine diameter
❑ the changes in uterine echogenicity and size are not sufficiently specific to allow the anticipation of ovulation time
❑ the echotexture returns to a homogeneous nature during metoestrus (dioestrus)
❑ uterine transverse section diameter continues to increase during early metoestrus

❑ uterine diameter increases in both pregnant and non-pregnant bitches
❑ pregnancy diagnosis requires the detection of fluid-filled (anechoic) conceptuses (see 12.9)

The normal ovary

❑ ovaries are difficult to examine due to their small size and superficial location
❑ during anoestrus the ovaries are located adjacent to the caudal pole of the kidney close to the lateral abdominal wall
❑ during oestrus they are often located more caudally and ventrally
❑ during anoestrus the ovaries of the bitch are less than 1.5 × 1.0 × 0.8 cm in size, and are relatively homogeneous
❑ at the onset of pro-oestrus small fluid filled anechoic follicles may be detected within the ovarian stroma
❑ when first imaged the internal diameter of follicles is between 1 and 2 mm
❑ follicles enlarge during pro-oestrus and become less spherical in outline
❑ the maximum follicular diameter is usually attained 1 day after the surge of plasma LH, i.e. the day before ovulation
❑ anechoic follicles are replaced by hypoechoic structures (presumably early corpora lutea) between 1 and 3 days after the surge of plasma LH; however, these structures are present only transiently, before being replaced by anechoic structures with 2 mm thick hypoechoic walls
❑ luteal structures are most commonly cavitated during early metoestrus (dioestrus)
❑ the time of ovulation is difficult to demonstrate without repeated examination of the bitch
❑ the detection of ovulation with ultrasound has limited value, especially when compared with more simple techniques such as vaginal cytology and measurement of plasma progesterone concentration (Fig. 4.3)

[handwritten: "Best" visualised d∝t to ovulation]
[handwritten: -daily u/s needed for procedure to be of clin. value]

4.9 MEASUREMENT OF PLASMA HORMONES (see Fig. 3.1)

❑ measurement of the plasma concentrations of the steroid hormones may be useful for estimating the stage of the oestrous cycle
❑ conventionally hormone concentrations are measured by radioimmunoassay; however
  (a) these are often costly
  (b) samples are often only assayed in batches
  (c) there is often a delay in receiving the results
❑ hormone concentrations may be accurately measured using enzyme-linked immunosorbent assay (ELISA) techniques:
  (a) these can be performed in the practice laboratory
  (b) results may usually be obtained within 1 hour of sample collection
❑ in the UK both quantative and qualitative ELISA methods are available for the assessment of progesterone concentration:

[handwritten: Hormone determination useful for: • breeding management • Ovarian remnant syndrome diag • mismating monitoring • follicular cyst diag • luteal cyst diag]
[handwritten: poor accuracy of ELISA kits]

(a)

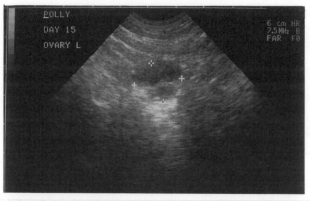

(b)

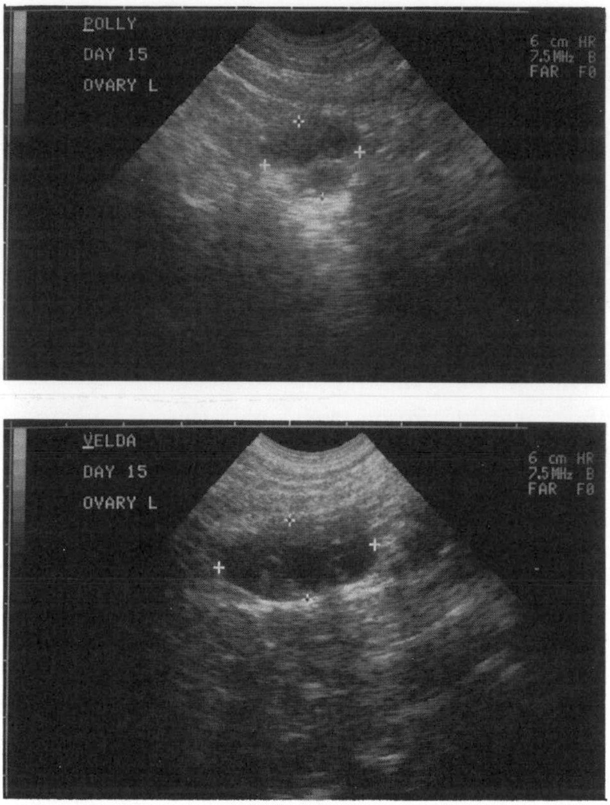

Handwritten note (left margin, top): when fbred by accident, give prostaglandins ~ 10 days after end of heat, check progesterone levels → should go down ~ 2 days.

Fig. 4.3 Ultrasound image of a bitch ovary: (a) during oestrus, three small circular anechoic follicles are present; (b) during early metoestrus (dioestrus), three thick walled anechoic corpora lutea are present (5.0 MHz transducer, scale in centimetres).

(a) quantitative techniques require the use of a plate reader and plotting of a standard curve for known progesterone standards

(b) qualitative techniques allow the estimation of progesterone concentration by comparison of a colour change with known progesterone standards

Plasma (serum) progesterone concentration

Handwritten note (left margin): High progesterone when no longer in heat

☐ progesterone is produced solely by the pre-ovulatory follicle and the corpus luteum in the bitch
☐ progesterone concentrations increase immediately before ovulation
☐ progesterone concentrations peak approximately 10–15 days after ovulation
☐ serial monitoring of plasma progesterone therefore allows:
    (a) anticipation of ovulation
    (b) confirmation of ovulation
    (c) detection of the fertilization period (see Chapter 11)
☐ values decrease slowly throughout the luteal phase

Handwritten note (left margin, bottom): ↑ P4 before ovulation

Handwritten note (bottom): "ovary mah sensra" may have some adrenal production

❏ progesterone concentrations are similar in pregnancy and non-pregnancy (non-pregnant values are lower, but because of individual variation values cannot be used to diagnose pregnancy or non-pregnancy)
❏ the non-pregnant luteal phase lasts approximately 68 days from ovulation
❏ the pregnant luteal phase lasts approximately 63 days from ovulation
❏ there is a sudden decrease in progesterone 24–36 hours before parturition

Interpretation

Stage of cycle	Progesterone concentration
Anoestrus	Basal – less than 1.0 ng/ml (less than 3.0 nmol/l)
Pro-oestrus	Basal – less than 1.0 ng/ml (less than 3.0 nmol/l)
Oestrus	Basal – less than 1.0 ng/ml (less than 3.0 nmol/l)
Day of LH surge	Intermediate – 2.0 ng/ml (6.5 nmol/l)
Day of ovulation	Intermediate – 5.0 ng/ml (15 nmol/l)
End of fertilization period	High – 8.0 to 10.0 ng/ml (25.0 to 32.0 nmol/l)
Non-pregnant luteal phase	High early, intermediate later
Pregnant luteal phase	High early, intermediate later

[handwritten margin note: DO NOT LEARN]

Plasma (serum) oestrogen concentration

[handwritten note: levels ↑ during estrus]

❏ oestrogen concentrations during the majority of anoestrus are low
❏ concentrations increase in late anoestrus and throughout pro-oestrus
❏ peak values are reached during late pro-oestrus or early oestrus, approximately 2 days before the LH surge
❏ concentrations are low at the time of ovulation
❏ concentrations during oestrus may therefore be high or low depending upon when a sample is taken in relation to ovulation
❏ oestrogen concentrations increase during the late non-pregnant and late pregnant luteal phase
❏ measurement of resting plasma oestrogen concentration has little clinical indication in the female

[handwritten margin note: levels low @ ovulation]

Plasma (serum) luteinizing hormone (LH) concentration

❏ concentrations of LH increase from 1 month before ovulation
❏ there is a large pre-ovulatory LH surge (values increase by 20 to 40 times)
❏ the pre-ovulatory surge occurs approximately 1–2 days after peak values of oestrogen are reached
❏ the pre-ovulatory surge lasts 24–72 hours
❏ serial sampling and the detection of the LH surge therefore allows:
(a) anticipation of ovulation
(b) detection of the fertilization period (see Chapter 11)
❏ LH is, however, only reliably measured by radioimmunoassay at present
❏ LH is luteotrophic and is elevated similarly in the pregnant and non-pregnant luteal phase

[handwritten margin notes: LH peak = Day 0 of cycle; ovulation = D2; fertilization - days 4-6; whelping = D64]

[handwritten note at bottom: No practical test for LH. Day 0 determines indirectly c̄ P4 serum level testing (2ng)]

4.10 BACTERIAL EXAMINATION OF THE FEMALE REPRODUCTIVE TRACT

Vestibule and caudal vagina

- have a normal bacterial flora — *usually mixed*
- this changes daily
- many species of bacteria are present, including haemolytic streptococci, other streptococci, staphylococci *Escherichia coli*, and many others
- ureoplasmata and mycoplasmata are also normal
- there is usually a mixed flora, with 2–5 species present
- the incidence of anaerobic bacteria is not well documented
- *Pseudomonas* spp. are not commonly isolated from normal bitches
- there is no correlation between the numbers of organisms cultured and those seen in vaginal smears; this suggests that some stained bacteria may be dead or are anaerobes

no correlation btwn culture results & fertility problems

Cranial vagina *(usually lower bact #)*

- there is little information on the flora of the cranial vagina and cervix because no reliable sampling method has been devised
- vagino-cervical defence mechanisms, i.e. mucus production with discharge to the vulva and neutrophil mobilization, may normally discourage bacterial colonization of the cranial vagina

due to this

- vaginal culture one of the most abused procedures

Uterus

- the uterus is usually thought to be bacteriologically sterile when healthy
- however:
  (a) one study has isolated organisms from apparently normal uteri
  (b) it seems likely that the vaginal flora will be introduced into the uterus with the ejaculate during coitus
  (c) in post-partum metritis and pyometra bacteria of vaginal origin appear to be capable of contributing to the disease process
- it is possible to collect samples from the uterus using endoscopic techniques; however, these are liable to contamination from the cranial vagina and results should be interpreted cautiously

may contain contaminants if not collected via laparotomy

DO NOT EXPECT A ⊘ RESULT !!!

Interpretation of vaginal bacteriology

- a positive culture should result in ↑ WBCs

- most swab samples are taken from the vestibule
- they should therefore be expected to contain bacteria
- there is no evidence that colonization of the caudal vagina and vestibule by bacteria is a sign of disease
- there is no evidence of coital influence on the vestibular bacterial flora
- withholding mating because of isolation of β-haemolytic streptococci from the vestibule seems unnecessary
- consideration should be given to the probability that the dog has a resident

cultures by themselves are not diagnostic - need to c̄ complete c̄ cytology & pe

Brucellosis swab = diagnostic
↳ only true pathogen in UGT

penile flora (see 15.2) which may be enhanced by contact between the penis and the bitch's coat, anus, etc., before intromission
- ❏ the isolation of a single species of bacterium (pure culture) from the tract may be more significant than a mixed culture
- ❏ venereal spread of organisms other than bacteria is possible, but has not been confirmed
- ❏ much more research is necessary before the possible role of bacteria in bitch infertility can be elucidated
- ❏ the only known bacterial venereal pathogen in the dog is *Brucella canis*
- ❏ routine bacteriological screening in the clinically normal bitch is pointless

4.11 ENDOCRINOLOGICAL STIMULATION TESTS

- ❏ measurement of basal hormone concentrations is not always diagnostic
- ❏ hormone stimulation tests may be useful to confirm the presence of a functional pituitary–ovarian interaction (the gonadotrophin-releasing hormone (GnRH) stimulation test)
- ❏ hormone stimulation tests may be useful to confirm the presence of functional ovarian tissue (the human chorionic gonadotrophin (hCG) stimulation test)

The gonadotrophin releasing hormone (GnRH) stimulation test

- ❏ a plasma (serum) sample is collected and assayed for LH and oestrogen concentration
- ❏ a GnRH analogue is injected intravenously (0.01 µg/kg buserelin) and a second sample is assayed for LH and oestrogen concentration 60 minutes later
- ❏ a significant increase in LH concentration indicates the presence of a functional pituitary gland
- ❏ a significant increase in oestrogen concentration indicates the presence of a functional pituitary gland and ovary (the test may be used to confirm the presence or absence of ovarian tissue in bitches with an unknown reproductive history)

The human chorionic gonadotrophin (hCG) stimulation test

- ❏ hCG is used rather than LH because the latter is not commercially available
- ❏ hCG is principally LH-like in activity
- ❏ a plasma (serum) sample is collected and assayed for oestrogen concentration
- ❏ hCG is injected intravenously (50 IU/kg) and a second sample is assayed for oestrogen concentration 60 minutes later
- ❏ a significant increase in oestrogen concentration indicates the presence of functional ovarian tissue (the test may be used to confirm the presence or absence of ovarian tissue in bitches with an unknown reproductive history)

4.12 LAPAROSCOPY AND LAPAROTOMY

❏ laparoscopy and laparotomy are not widely performed for the investigation of reproductive tract disease

may be useful in diagnosing cystic endometrial hypertrophy (CEH)

❏ both techniques may be useful when other diagnostic tools have failed
❏ these techniques enable abnormalities of the tubular genital tract to be diagnosed

4.13 KARYOTYPING

❏ may be useful in certain cases of infertility
❏ there are a limited number of institutions offering this service
❏ requires collection of blood into EDTA anticoagulant and rapid transport to the laboratory
❏ chromosomes are examined from metaphase spreads following culture

ovary difficult to evaluate due to ovarian bursa

— may be useful w/ cases of intersex cases w/o abnormalities of ext. genitalia

— routine karyotyping in unexplained infertility of limited use

5 Anatomy of the Dog's Reproductive Tract

5.1 PREPUCE

- ❏ completely covers the non-erect penis
- ❏ the outside is covered by skin, the inside by a mucous membrane which is continuous with the mucosa of the penis at the base of the *glans penis*

5.2 PENIS

- ❏ the *glans penis* starts at the attachment to the inner lining of the prepuce and is composed of:
  (a) the proximal *bulbus glandis* – in the non-erect state this is hardly discernible; when the penis is erect the bulbus glandis becomes a roughly spherical swelling which is responsible for locking the penis into the bitch's vagina during coitus (see 8.3)
  (b) the *pars longa glandis* comprises the distal three-quarters of the glans and terminates in the opening of the urethra
- ❏ the *os penis* is a bone which is surrounded by the glans penis; it is broad proximally and narrower distally and has a ventral groove which houses the urethra

5.3 TESTES (Fig. 5.1)

- ❏ pass through the inguinal canal 4 days after birth
- ❏ reach their scrotal location by 4–6 weeks and usually earlier
- ❏ are roughly ovoid in shape
- ❏ the long axis of the testis lies longitudinally
- ❏ the bulk of the testis is composed of *seminiferous tubules*, in which spermatozoa are produced by the process of *spermatogenesis*
- ❏ the seminiferous tubules are supported by a network of fibrous tissue called the *mediastinum testis*
- ❏ the seminiferous tubules empty into a collecting system, the *rete testis*, which conducts spermatozoa away from the testis and into the epididymis

5.4 EPIDIDYMIS

- ❏ this is a very long tube which is coiled tightly onto itself to form a structure which can be described as having a head, body and tail

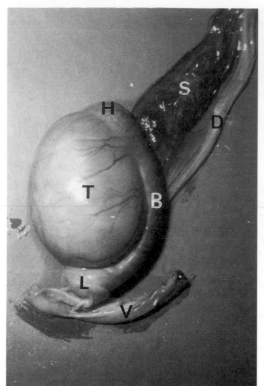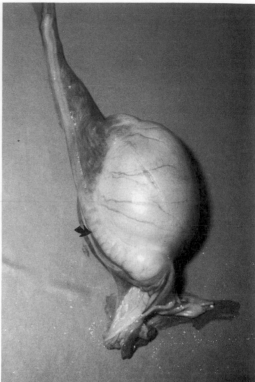

Fig. 5.1 Testis and adnexa: (a) lateral view; testis (T), head (H), body (B) and tail (L) of epididymis, spermatic cord (S) and ductus deferens (D). The tail of the epididymis is attached to the tunica vaginalis propria (V) by the ligament of the tail of the epididymis; (b) medial view; the ductus deferens is convoluted proximally (arrowed).

- ❏ during their passage through the epididymis spermatozoa become mature; in the dog this takes about 14 days
- ❏ the head (caput) of the epididymis is on the cranio-lateral border of the testis and is not readily palpable
- ❏ the body (corpus) of the epididymis is on the dorso-lateral surface of the testis and cannot be palpated
- ❏ the tail (cauda) of the epididymis is on the dorso-caudal pole of the testis; it is readily palpable in the normal animal as a firm 'pea-sized' protuberance which does not appear to be contiguous with the body
- ❏ the epididymis now continues as a straight tube which contains mature spermatozoa and is called the *ductus (vas) deferens*

5.5   DUCTUS DEFERENS (VAS DEFERENS)

- ❏ this duct conveys spermatozoa from the epididymis to the urethra
- ❏ it runs into the abdomen in the spermatic cord

❏ in the abdomen it passes cranial to the ureter and empties into the urethra in the cranial prostate gland
❏ the ducti (vasa) deferentia are about 1 mm in diameter, pale coloured and 'wiry' – they arc good landmarks for locating abdominal testes during surgery (see 27.9)

5.6   SPERMATIC CORD

❏ this is a bundle of various tissues which runs between the testis and the abdominal wall
❏ it has four main components:
(a) the *ductus deferens*
(b) the *cremaster muscle:* this ariscs from thc internal abdominal oblique muscle near the external inguinal ring and is attached to the vaginal tunic at the level of the testis; it can vary the distance between the testis and abdominal wall, thus regulating testis temperature
(c) thc *spermatic (testicular) artery:* this conveys blood from the aorta to the testis and runs through the *pampiniform plexus*
(d) the *spermatic (testicular) vein:* this conducts blood from the testis to the *vena cava;* in the spermatic cord the vein divides into a complex of small veins (thc *pampiniform plexus*) which surrounds the spermatic artery. The cool blood returning from the testicle reduces the temperature of the arterial blood to ensure that the testis does not become overheated
NB: a special musclc in thc scrotal skin, thc *dartos,* can also regulate the proximity of the testes to the body wall and thus influence their temperature

5.7   INGUINAL CANAL

❏ the spermatic vessels and the ductus deferens pass into the abdomen through a narrow space in the muscles of the abdominal wall – the inguinal canal
❏ occasionally this canal is wide enough to allow the escape of some abdominal contents to form an inguinal hernia; this may also happen in the bitch (see 15.8 and 19.6)
❏ close to the inguinal canal is the inguinal lymph node that may become enlarged when there is testicular pathology

5.8   PROSTATE GLAND

❏ this is the only accessory gland in the male dog
❏ it is a bilobed structure situated at the pelvic inlet
❏ the urethra passes through the gland before it reaches the base of the penis
❏ the ducti (vasa) deferentia also pass through a small amount of the cranial aspect of the gland before they enter the urethra dorsally
❏ the gland produces a clear secretion which is expelled into the urethra; this secretion is the first and third fractions of the ejaculate (see 6.6)
❏ prostatic fluid is bacteriocidal

❑ the position and size of the gland are very variable
❑ the gland normally increases in size with advancing age; increase in size is usually accompanied by a more abdominal position
❑ the gland is prone to pathological changes which also cause an increase in size; it is often difficult to decide whether or not abnormal growth has occurred (see 15.7)

5.9   URETHRA

❑ this tube has the function of conveying both urine and semen to the tip of the penis
❑ it originates at the bladder neck and travels caudally on the floor of the pelvis through the prostate gland; here the ducti deferentia open into its dorsal surface
❑ at the caudal limit of the ischium the urethra enters the penis and runs on its caudo-ventral aspect eventually entering the ventral groove of the os penis

6 Reproductive Physiology of the Dog

6.1 SPERMATOGENESIS

❏ this is the complicated process by which spermatozoa are produced, and it occurs in the seminiferous tubules of the testes

❏ cells called *spermatogonia* which are the precursors of spermatozoa divide in the usual manner (mitosis) to produce very many *spermatocytes*

❏ spermatocytes then divide by meiosis in which the normal number of chromosomes in the resulting cells is halved to 39 and the genetic material derived from the individual's parents is mixed

❏ the resulting cells are called spermatids and are described as being *haploid* (half the usual number of chromosomes – cells with 78 chromosomes are said to be *diploid*; this includes the two sex chromosomes)

❏ spermatids change into spermatozoa by a complex rearrangement of organelles; basically the nucleus becomes the sperm head, the Golgi apparatus forms the acrosome, and the mitochondria and centrioles are involved in the development of the mid piece and tail (see 9.5)

❏ most of the cytoplasm is left in the *Sertoli cells* which are situated on the basement membrane of the seminiferous tubule; they regulate the metamorphosis from spermatid to spermatozoon

❏ spermatogenesis starts at 4 months of age but spermatozoa do not appear in the ejaculate until approximately 10–12 months

6.2 TEMPERATURE CONTROL

❏ spermatogenesis cannot occur at normal body temperature in most mammals

❏ the mechanisms which keep the dog's testes cooler than the rest of the body have been mentioned in Chapter 5 and are:

(a) the testes are housed outside the body in the scrotal sac

(b) the cremaster muscle can influence the distance between the body and testis

(c) the *dartos muscle* in the scrotal wall can influence the size of the scrotum and thus the position of the testes

(d) the arrangement of the blood vessels in the spermatic cord allows cooling of arterial blood by the venous return in the pampiniform plexus (see 5.6)

❏ conditions which cause elevated body temperature, e.g. fever and heat stroke, may not be compensated for by these mechanisms and can impair spermatogenesis

❏ obesity may also reduce testicular cooling

6.3   SPERMATOZOAL TRANSPORT

❏ spermatozoa enter the caput epididymis in an immature state; they have a droplet of residual cytoplasm at the neck called a proximal cytoplasmic drop (see 9.5) which is sometimes incorrectly called the 'protoplasmic' droplet

❏ during the passage of spermatozoa along the epididymis, which is presumably caused by the constant production of more spermatozoa from the testis, the cells mature

❏ on entry into the ductus deferens the cytoplasmic droplet has moved to the distal end of the mid piece or become detached from the spermatozoon, which is now considered to be mature

❏ factors which might influence the speed of movement along the ductus deferens are unknown

❏ spermatozoa which are not voided by ejaculation are thought to be forced to the opening of the ductus deferens and into the urethra by the build-up of cells behind them; they may then travel cranially to the bladder and are expelled in urine

❏ during ejaculation spermatozoa are actively expelled from the ductus deferens into the urethra

❏ there is little evidence to support the concept that the ejaculate from an infrequently 'used' stud dog will contain an abnormally high number of abnormal spermatozoa

❏ the spermatogenic cycle, i.e. from division of spermatogonia to the appearance of spermatozoa in the ejaculate, takes 8 weeks; for two of these weeks the spermatozoa are maturing in the epididymis

6.4   PROSTATE GLAND

❏ produces the first and third fractions of the dog's ejaculate (see 9.5)

❏ the function of the first fraction is probably to flush the urethra clear of any urine or cellular debris

❏ the function of the third fraction of the ejaculate is probably to wash the sperm-rich second fraction from the cranial vagina into the uterus of the bitch

❏ disease of the prostate (15.7) may affect fertility because:
(a) blood can affect spermatozoal viability in some cases but this is unlikely in dogs
(b) the effect of prostatic infection (and subsequent changes in the nature of the prostatic fluid) on spermatozoal function is unknown
(c) drugs used to reduce prostatic size (oestrogens and progestogens) may also inhibit spermatogenesis (see 24.1 and 24.2)

❏ surprisingly, spermatozoa incubated *in vitro* in prostatic fluid are less viable than those in semen extenders; it seems therefore that prostatic fluid *per se* is not supportive of spermatozoal function

6.5 ERECTION

- ❏ factors which stimulate erection in most animals are the smell of a female in oestrus and association between routine and coitus
- ❏ the pathways by which these stimuli initiate erection are probably neural, but are not completely understood
- ❏ erection is tumescence (swelling and turgidity) of the penis due to an accumulation of blood in its tissues caused by constriction of venous return
- ❏ in dogs only slight erection occurs before coitus; intromission is facilitated by the rigidity afforded by the os penis and total erection then occurs to ensure that the penis becomes 'locked' into the female genital tract (see 8.3)
- ❏ it is only after the erection has subsided that the dog and bitch can subsequently part

6.6 EJACULATION

- ❏ contractions of the urethral muscle force fluids from the ducti deferentia and prostate gland into and along the urethra

First fraction

- ❏ during initial sexual excitement the first fraction of the ejaculate is voided
- ❏ this varies in volume but is usually approximately 0.5–2.0 ml
- ❏ it may be ejaculated while the dog is thrusting during attempts to introduce his penis into the bitch's vagina, or may be voided after intromission
- ❏ it originates from the prostate gland and may have the function of washing the urethra clear of urine

Second fraction

- ❏ the second fraction is usually ejaculated after intromission when thrusting ceases
- ❏ this is the sperm-rich portion of the ejaculate and is usually 0.5–1.0 ml in volume
- ❏ it originates from the ducti deferentia and is deposited into the anterior half of the vagina during completion of the dog's erection
- ❏ during and soon after ejaculation of this fraction, the dog instinctively wants to 'turn' (see 8.3)

Third fraction

- ❏ the third fraction originates from the prostate gland
- ❏ it is usually voided whilst the dogs are standing tail to tail in the 'tie' position
- ❏ the volume may approach 15–20 ml in large breeds and is probably related to the length of the 'tie'

❏ the function of this fraction is thought to be that of washing the spermatozoa forward into the uterus; however, the effect of third fraction on spermatozoa may not always be favourable (see 6.4)

❏ termination of ejaculation is followed by detumescence of the penis and its withdrawal

7 Endocrinology of Reproduction in the Dog

7.1 GONADOTROPHIN RELEASING HORMONE (GnRH) (see 3.1)

❑ produced in the hypothalamus (at the base of the brain) and conveyed to the anterior pituitary gland via a specialized system of blood vessels
❑ responsible for selectively causing release of follicle stimulating hormone (FSH) and luteinizing hormone (LH) from the anterior pituitary gland
❑ secretion is episodic
❑ pulsatile rather than continuous secretion is necessary for the induction and maintenance of normal gonadotrophin release

7.2 FOLLICLE STIMULATING HORMONE (FSH)

❑ FSH release is slow and gradual after GnRH stimulation
❑ FSH binds to Sertoli cells and spermatogonia
❑ binding results in the production of a variety of proteins that may be important in regulating spermatogenesis via androgen binding protein and transferrin
❑ feedback control of FSH is via the gonadal peptide inhibin, and possibly modulation of Leydig cell function

7.3 LUTEINIZING HORMONE (LH) OR INTERSTITIAL CELL STIMULATING HORMONE (ICSH)

❑ LH release is immediate but transient after GnRH stimulation
❑ plasma concentrations increase and return to basal within 60 minutes
❑ LH binds to Leydig cells of the testis
❑ LH stimulates testicular steroidogenesis
❑ a rise in plasma LH is followed by a rise of plasma testosterone within 60 minutes

7.4 ANDROGENS (testosterone and dihydrotestosterone)

❑ produced by cells in the testis which form little islands between the seminiferous tubules; these are interstitial cells or Leydig cells
❑ testosterone secretion occurs both locally within the testis and into the peripheral circulation
❑ most testosterone secreted into the plasma is bound to plasma proteins

❑ peripheral testosterone is necessary for the development and maintenance of secondary sexual characteristics, maintenance of sexual behaviour, and negative feedback regulation of gonadotrophin secretion

❑ high intra-testicular testosterone concentrations are maintained within the seminiferous tubules by binding to androgen binding protein

❑ high local testosterone concentrations are important for the initiation and maintenance of spermatogenesis

❑ testosterone and its active metabolites oestradiol and dihydrotestosterone exert a profound feedback effect on FSH and LH

❑ ectopic testes (e.g. in cryptorchids; see 15.3) still produce androgens

❑ in mature dogs plasma testosterone concentrations vary between 0.5 and 5.0 ng/ml; there is a great deal of variation throughout the day in an individual dog, so that assay of a single sample is of little value

❑ in castrated dogs, values are consistently below 200 pg/ml

❑ in order to diagnose the presence of an unidentified ectopic testis a human chorionic gonadotrophin (hCG) stimulation test can be performed (see 4.11); a rise in testosterone concentration indicates the presence of testicular tissue

7.5   INHIBIN

❑ this is a hormone produced by the Sertoli cells of the testis and inhibits the release of FSH

❑ its existence in the dog has not been proven

7.6   ACTIVINS

❑ there is increasing evidence that the Sertoli cells produce other substances, termed activins, that have a stimulatory effect upon FSH secretion

8 Mating (Coitus)

8.1 PLANNING THE MATING

- ❏ in selecting a stud dog for a bitch, the following factors should be considered:
  - (a) desirability of conformation and temperament
  - (b) distance to be travelled
  - (c) cost of stud fee
  - (d) freedom from inherited diseases
  - (e) pedigree related to that of the bitch
  - (f) potential value of puppies for showing, racing, etc.
  - (g) availability, i.e. popularity
- ❏ a contract with the stud dog owner is best written and signed and should contain details of the stud fee, whether it is payable if the bitch does not conceive, whether the bitch has a free return if she does not conceive and whether the stud dog owner has the 'pick' of the litter of pups
- ❏ the help of an experienced dog breeder should be sought if bitch and dog owner are novices
- ❏ inform the dog owner when the first signs of pro-oestrus are noted in the bitch

8.2 TIMING

- ❏ most bitches are mated 10–12 days after the beginning of pro-oestrus
- ❏ this usually gives sastisfactory results even if the bitch is not ovulating at this time because:
  - (a) sperm from a fertile dog can survive for up to 7 days in the bitch, so that matings before ovulation can be fertile
  - (b) ova are not ready to be fertilized until 3 days after ovulation, so that matings after ovulation may be fertile (see 11.3)
- ❏ however, an inappropriate mating time is the most common cause of alleged infertility in the bitch (see 10.1)
- ❏ repeated matings 24–48 hours apart increase the likelihood of conception
- ❏ help in detecting ovulation time may be required when:
  - (a) bitches ovulate much earlier or later than average (see 2.4)
  - (b) artificial insemination is being used (see 22.10)
  - (c) a dog with poor semen quality is being used; repeated matings may still be advantageous (see 21.6)
  - (d) a bitch is 'shy' and may need to be restrained during mating
- ❏ ovulation time can be detected using vaginal endoscopy, vaginal cytology, or by measuring blood progesterone concentrations (see 3.5)

8.3   NORMAL COITAL BEHAVIOUR

Foreplay

❑   if dog and bitch are unrestrained a variable amount of sniffing, jumping and playing occurs, during which the dog, particularly if he is inexperienced, will mount the bitch in various inappropriate positions
❑   during this time first fraction may be ejaculated (see 6.6)
❑   if the bitch is cooperative she will eventually stand still to allow the dog to mount her from behind, and she will raise her tail to one side and lift her vulva to facilitate intromission
❑   some bitches may need to be held by the head and be muzzled in order to prevent the risk of the dogs biting each other, or an aggressive bitch frightening an inexperienced dog

Intromission

❑   once the dog has mounted he will commence thrusting movements in order to try to achieve intromission; at this time erection is only slight and rigidity is afforded by the os penis (see 5.2)
❑   the fore limbs of the dog grip the bitch tightly in front of her pelvis
❑   on gaining intromission more purposeful thrusts ensure that the whole glans penis is inserted; the dog's pelvis is forced very close to the bitch at this stage, and his lower back is almost vertical
❑   erection starts after full intromission, and the dog ejaculates the second, sperm-rich fraction at this time

The tie

❑   once full erection has occurred the dog instinctively wants to dismount
❑   by placing both front feet to one side of the bitch, the back leg on the opposite side is left in the air
❑   the dog lifts this leg over the bitch's back whilst turning round
❑   this causes the penis, proximal to the os penis, to bend laterally through 180°
❑   if the dog has a full erection, his penis will not leave the bitch's vagina
❑   the dog is still able to complete ejaculation of the third fraction, even though the urethra is bent
❑   bending of the penis may help to prevent escape of blood from the glans and thus maintain erection
NB: in some breeds, e.g. greyhounds, a complete turn is not usually allowed by the handler; this does not seem to affect fertility, but is an inappropriate strategy

8.4   FACTORS PREVENTING NORMAL MATING (see 18.6 and Chapter 21)

Psychological factors

Most dogs know instinctively how to copulate but on occasion may not be able to because of:

❏   a difference in sexual experience; an experienced stud may frighten a virgin bitch or vice versa
❏   fear of human disapproval; this is particularly true of male dogs which have previously been reprimanded for displaying sexual interest
❏   unfamiliarity with the venue; because the dog takes the more active role in coitus the bitch is usually taken to the dog's residence in order to avoid this problem
❏   overfamiliarity; sometimes dogs and bitches kept together all the time will not copulate
❏   humanization: particularly bitches, when kept in houses and rarely exposed to other dogs, appear to resent the approach of another dog as if it were 'abnormal'
❏   lack of libido: in male dogs this may be similar to the previously mentioned problem in the bitch. The cause could also be some of the other afore-mentioned psychological factors
❏   diagnosis and therapy are difficult:
     (a) measurement of circulating testosterone concentrations is not diagnostic because of the large variation throughout the day in the normal dog
     (b) administration of human chorionic gonadotrophin (hCG) may increase testosterone production but is not therapeutic
     (c) administration of testosterone is also not therapeutic and may cause aggression and impaired spermatogenesis (due to inhibition of release of pituitary gonadotrophins)
     (d) thyroid replacement therapy may improve libido but such regimes have not been properly evaluated

Physical factors

❏   dogs with obvious limb deformities and musculo-skeletal lesions may have problems achieving a position compatible with intromission; they should not be used for breeding if their condition is inherited
❏   subtle lumbar or lumbo-socral lesions may prevent dogs from mating, even though there is no evidence of pain in other everyday activities
❏   bitches may require help to hold up heavy dogs
❏   dogs with prostatic disease may show signs of pain during or after ejaculation (see 15.7)
❏   non-steroidal anti-inflammatory drugs may reduce musculo-skeletal pain and are not known to be detrimental to semen
NB: it may be difficult to ascertain whether a dog's reluctance to copulate is due to physical or psychological factors

Failure to tie

❏   after intromission the tie may not occur due to both dog and bitch factors
❏   if ejaculation of the second fraction has occurred, the bitch may still conceive, although fertility is not thought to be good
❏   the effect of the length of the tie on fertility is not known, although many breeders feel that a long tie enhances the chance of conception

9 Clinical Examination of the Dog's Reproductive Tract

9.1 BASIC EXAMINATION OF THE REPRODUCTIVE TRACT

This consists of:

❏ visual examination of the prepuce and penis
❏ palpation of the scrotum
❏ semen collection and evaluation
❏ real-time ultrasonographic imaging
❏ measurement of plasma hormone concentrations
❏ observation of mating behaviour

9.2 ADDITIONAL TECHNIQUES THAT MAY BE CONSIDERED

These include:

❏ bacterial examination of the reproductive tract
❏ testicular biopsy
❏ testicular fine-needle aspiration
❏ prostatic biopsy
❏ prostatic massage/urethral flushing
❏ endocrinological stimulation tests
❏ karyotyping

9.3 VISUAL EXAMINATION OF THE PENIS AND PREPUCE

❏ best initially examined in the absence of the bitch
❏ a mucopurulent discharge from the prepuce is common and *normal*
❏ the prepuce should cover the length of the penis
❏ multiple lymphoid nodules are frequently found at the base of the penis on the *bulbus glandis*
❏ examination should also be performed on the erect penis after semen collection

9.4 PALPATION OF THE SCROTUM

❏ the scrotal skin should have no lesions
❏ the testes should be freely mobile within the scrotum
❏ testes should be similarly sized and have reasonable tone
❏ the tail of the epididymides should be carefully palpated

9.5   SEMEN COLLECTION AND EVALUATION

Reasons for semen evaluation

- ❏ to confirm normal spermatogenesis in a young dog before starting a stud career
- ❏ to monitor semen quality during the career of a stud dog
- ❏ to ensure suitable semen quality in an aged dog
- ❏ as part of any artificial insemination programme
- ❏ prior to semen preservation
- ❏ in cases of infertility where the dog may be implicated
- ❏ to monitor semen production after illness or drug therapy
- ❏ to investigate the effect of prostatic disease on semen quality

Collection prerequisites

Have a bitch in late pro-oestrus or oestrus present

- ❏ inexperienced dogs are otherwise unlikely to ejaculate
- ❏ the dog is usually taken to a venue strange to him where he is not used to 'working', which may inhibit even an experienced dog
- ❏ slippery floors or personnel wearing white coats may 'put the dog off'
- ❏ failure to collect a sample may upset the dog (and cause extra expense)

NB: vaginal secretion on swabs from oestrous bitches may be stored frozen and used to stimulate otherwise reluctant dogs – the thawed swab is held in front of the dog's nose. The dog pheromone methyl-*p*-hydoxybenzoate is available commercially in the USA

Select an appropriate procedure

- ❏ owners or handlers who are normally present when the dog mates may encourage interest
- ❏ small breeds are often mated on a table with a suitable surface
- ❏ large breeds mate on the floor with various degrees of human guidance
- ❏ the ejaculate consists of three distinct fractions which, for proper evaluation, should be collected separately:

  first fraction: prostatic fluid

  second fraction: sperm-rich fluid

  third fraction: prostatic fluid

- ❏ techniques for collection should therefore enable the fractional nature to be recognized and collected

Collection procedure

Equipment required

❑ two or three glass or plastic funnels
❑ two or three glass or plastic test tubes
NB: plastic will not break, but because it is light in weight it can easily be dislodged from the hand by the dog's tail or leg
❑ a water bath, preferably maintained automatically at 37°C
❑ a test tube rack in the water bath
❑ microscope slides and cover slips
❑ ideally, a 'warm stage' which keeps a microscope slide at 37°C (a flat bottle filled with warm water may be used to stand the microscope slides on to keep them warm)
❑ pipettes
❑ nigrosin/eosin stain
❑ microscope with oil for high-power viewing
❑ Neubauer cell counting chamber
❑ equipment for 1/200 dilution of semen

Collection technique (Fig. 9.1) (see also 6.6)

❑ the bitch is adequately restrained by the head or neck
❑ the dog is allowed to sniff and lick at the bitch's vulva
❑ when the dog seems interested, and before he tries to mount, the penis is held (usually by the operator's right hand, from the dog's left side)
❑ if the bulbus glandis is swollen, the prepuce should be pushed backwards to expose the whole glans
❑ if the bulbus glandis is not swollen, to and fro movement of the prepuce should stimulate the initial erection
❑ if the bulbus glandis becomes too swollen it is not possible to protrude the glans penis from the sheath; the dog should be taken away from the bitch until his erection has subsided, or an attempt may be made to collect with the penis in the sheath – this may be uncomfortable for the dog
❑ after exposure of the bulbus glandis, the base of the glans penis is gripped between the thumb and fore finger; it may be held firmly or rhythmic contractions applied
❑ pressure on the base of the penis should stimulate further swelling of the bulbus glandis with or without thrusting movements of the dog
❑ apart from premature swelling of the bulbus glandis, a major problem in exposing the penis is in long haired breeds, and in small breeds where holding the penis is difficult
❑ during violent thrusting movements there is no point in trying to collect the ejaculate because it will be sperm-free first fraction
❑ if first fraction is collected, it will be seen to be clear
❑ after expulsion of the first fraction the second (sperm-rich and white) fraction

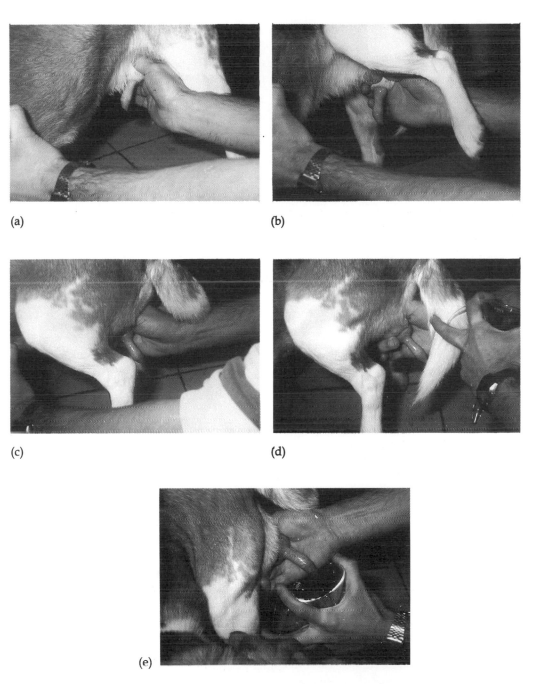

(a)   (b)

(c)   (d)

(e)

Fig. 9.1 Semen collection. (a) the prepuce is pushed backwards to expose the penis; (b) the dog lifts a hind leg, indicating his desire to 'turn'; (c) the penis is reflected backwards between the dog's legs; (d) continued pressure or rhythmic squeezing of the base of the bulbus glandis stimulates further erection to occur; (e) the penis is now fully erect and the ejaculate is being collected via a glass funnel.

is ejaculated in 4–10 urethral contractions; if possible this should be collected separately in the second test tube
- ❑ occasionally the volume of first fraction can approach 5 ml; if a nervous dog produces no sperm-rich fraction after this, a further collection should be considered
- ❑ after the sperm-rich fraction has been expelled, there may be several unproductive urethral contractions until the third fraction is ejaculated
- ❑ if the second fraction is very concentrated and of small volume, several 'spurts' of third fraction may be necessary to wash it from the collecting funnel and into the test tube
- ❑ the majority of the third fraction is either collected into the tube containing first fraction, or the dog is left to finish ejaculating onto the floor

Alternative collection techniques

Latex cone

- ❑ the test tube may be attached to a latex cone, which is placed over the dog's penis; this is not ideal because it is difficult to collect the fractions separately and because the latex may be toxic to sperm

Artificial vagina

- ❑ this is basically a cylindrical tube filled with warm water; it is totally inappropriate because:
  (a) it is unnecessary
  (b) it is complicated and cumbersome to use
  (c) it encourages prolonged contact between sperm and the latex liner which may cause complete immotility of the sperms

Evaluation of the sample (Fig. 9.2)

The sample is kept warm

This is important because:

- ❑ cooling of the sample causes a reduction in motility which will give a false impression of the quality of the sample
- ❑ a rapid decrease in temperature may cause 'cold-shock' damage to the spermatozoa; this rarely occurs in dog semen as it is relatively resistant to cold shock, and semen is usually collected at room temperature

Volume of the ejaculate

- ❑ this is measured in a graduated test tube, or by comparing such a tube with the sample tube
- ❑ the first fraction is normally 0.5–2.0 ml in volume
- ❑ the second fraction is normally 0.5–1.0 ml in volume

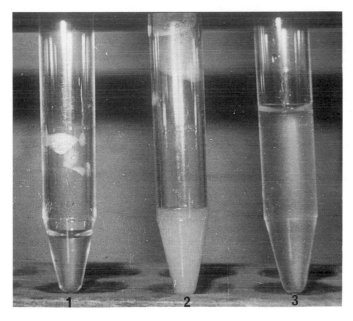

Fig. 9.2 The three fractions of the ejaculate. The second fraction is opaque and contains the spermatozoa.

❑ the third fraction is normally 15–20 ml in volume, but frequently this entire fraction is not collected

Colour of the ejaculate

❑ the first fraction is normally clear but may be contaminated with urine or cellular debris from the urethra
❑ the second fraction is normally white or creamy in colour
❑ the third fraction is normally clear
❑ occasionally there may be contamination with blood (especially the third fraction in middle-aged or old dogs), or other cells which will cause discolouration. If the sample is discoloured, examination of stained semen smears (e.g. using the modified Wright–Giemsa stain, Diff–Quik) may allow identification of contaminating cellular material such as red blood cells, or white blood cells

Spermatozoal concentration

This can be measured using:

❑ an *electronic counting chamber* which has been calibrated to count cells of this size. This is often inaccurate because sperm tails may lodge across the orifice of the device
❑ a *colorimeter* previously calibrated for dog semen. This has obvious inaccuracies

❏ a *haemocytometer* counting chamber (Fig. 9.3), after suitable dilution of the sample:
(a) a proportion of the semen is well mixed and is diluted 1 in 200 with distilled water containing a little detergent (the former kills spermatozoa and the latter prevents their clumping together)
(b) one drop is placed into the chamber which has a standard depth and a known grid engraved upon its surface. Counting the number of spermatozoa within the grid (known area therefore known volume) allows calculation of the original spermatozoal concentration. It is customary to count squares diagonally across the grid. Normal values are between 300×10^6 and 800×10^6/ml, but the total spermatozoal output is a more useful measure than concentration alone

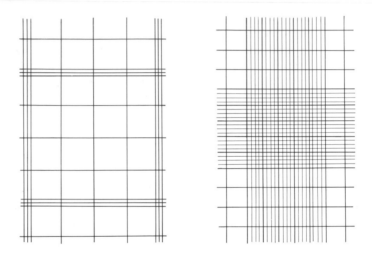

Fig. 9.3 Counting chamber grid. Spermatozoa are counted in five of the squares bounded by three parallel lines.

Total spermatozoal output

❏ this is a more meaningful measure than concentration or volume alone
❏ normal dogs produce between 300×10^6 and 1000×10^6 spermatozoa within each ejaculate

Percentage motility

❏ the vessel containing the semen must be placed immediately into a water bath at approximately 37°C to prevent cooling. A drop of semen is then placed onto a warmed microscope slide and covered with a cover slip. Evaluation at low temperatures will give erroneous results
❏ the sample should be assessed under low and high power magnification
❏ the assessment of motility is subjective, but the same observer can become very consistent

❏ samples should be assessed for the percentage of progressive motility. It is often easiest to categorize spermatozoal motility, using five groups:
category O: non-motile spermatozoa
category I: spermatozoa that are motile but not progressive
category II: spermatozoa that are motile but poorly progressive
category III: spermatozoa that are motile but moderately progressive
category IV: spermatozoa that are motile and rapidly progressive (swimming quickly in a forward direction)
Using these criteria normal dogs have more than 70% spermatozoa with category IV motility

❏ spermatozoa may be seen 'clumped' to each other and to other cells (epithelial cells or macrophages); the significance of this in the dog is not known but unless it affects the whole sample it is probably not a bad prognostic sign

❏ small round cells (erythrocytes or polymorphonuclear leucocytes) may be seen; preparation of a haematology smear may be necessary to distinguish between them (see p. 60)

❏ motility will decrease with time when the slide is left on the miscroscope stage (probably due to the effect of light and cooling)

Morphology

❏ this is the percentage of spermatozoa that conform to the shape accepted as normal for dog semen

❏ morphology can be examined in wet preparations, but in general fixation and staining of the sperm is necessary

❏ a variety of stains have been described including Giemsa

❏ a simple method may be used that allows spermatozoal morphology and membrane integrity to be established at the same time; this is called vital staining

❏ vital staining uses a simple stain, nigrosin–eosin that is best refrigerated between use

❏ the eosin is taken up by cells that were dead at the time of staining (damaged membranes), and they therefore appear pink

❏ the nigrosin provides a background stain so that the spermatozoa are silhouetted against it and their shape can be seen; nigrosin has a purple-blue colour

❏ spermatozoa that appear white are classified as live; these sperm have intact membranes which prevent the eosin from penetrating into the sperm

NB: the head of the spermatozoon is bilaterally flattened like a table tennis bat

Preparation of a sample for morphological examination with nigrosin–eosin

❏ place seven drops of nigrosin–eosin stain in a test tube and leave it to warm in the water bath for 2 minutes

❑ add one drop of semen (after mixing, as spermatozoa will have settled)
❑ immediately, with a fresh pipette, place one drop of stain–semen mixture onto a clean microscope slide
❑ using a second slide at an angle of 45°, draw a thin film of material across the first slide, as in preparing a smear for haematology
❑ allow the smear to dry (this is usually quite rapid)
❑ examine the slide under the × 100 objective lens using oil; if the spermatozoa are all overlying each other, another smear should be made using a larger volume of stain; if the spermatozoa are very sparse, another smear may be made using less stain
❑ the spermatozoa are seen in the smear silhouetted against the dark (nigrosin) background
❑ one hundred spermatozoa are examined and classified as either alive and normal, dead or abnormal (Fig. 9.4)

Classification of abnormal spermatozoa

❑ spermatozoal abnormalities can be classified into three categories:
(a) primary abnormalities occur during spermatogenesis
(b) secondary abnormalities occur during the epididymal phase of development
(c) tertiary abnormalities occur during collection and processing the sample
❑ classification of abnormalities may therefore be useful for elucidating their origin, and may provide information regarding the likely prognosis
❑ tables of primary, secondary and tertiary abnormalities are provided in standard textbooks
❑ the following are common abnormalities (also see pp. 57–59):
(a) head abnormalities
    lifted (oedematous) acrosomes
    knobbed acrosomes
    crater defect
(b) neck abnormalities
    bent neck
    broken neck
(c) mid piece abnormalities
    proximal cytoplasmic droplet
    neck tag (disrupted mitochondria)
(d) tail abnormalities
    distal cytoplasmic droplet (this is usually accepted as normal)
    bent tail
    coiled tail
(e) spermatozoa which are dead at the time of staining are penetrated by the eosin (pink)
NB: some nigrosin–eosin stains may cause tail abnormalities
❑ normal dogs will have more than 80% morphologically normal live spermatozoa within the ejaculate

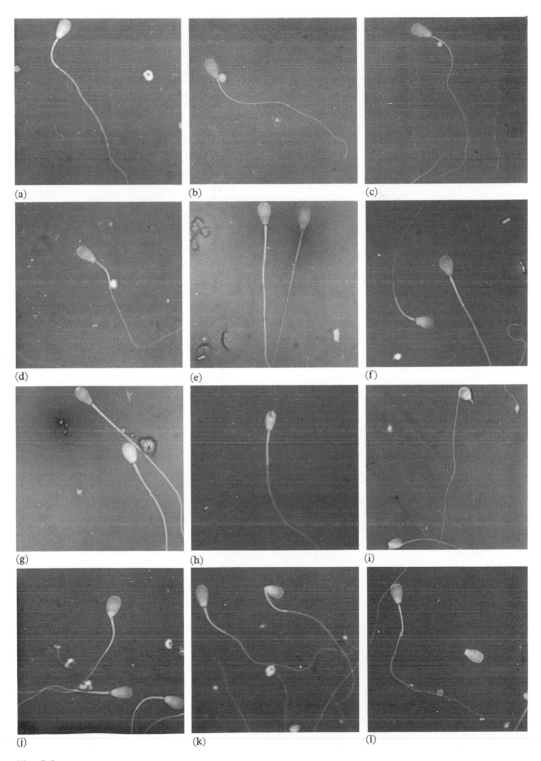

(a) (b) (c)

(d) (e) (f)

(g) (h) (i)

(j) (k) (l)

Fig. 9.4

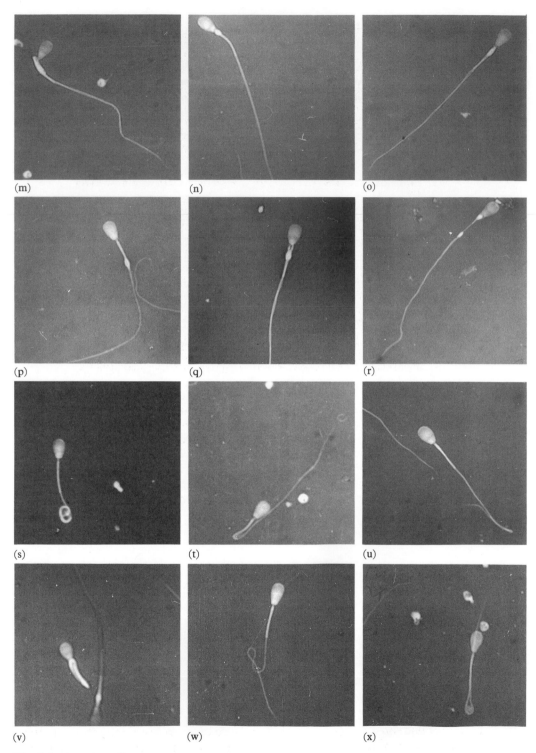

Fig. 9.4 (continued)

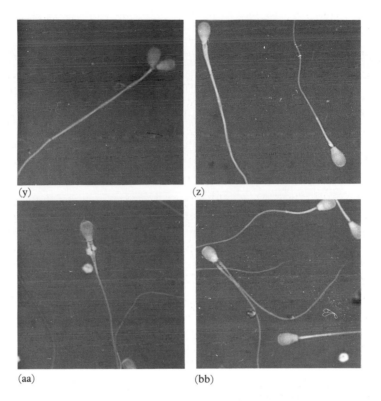

(y)   (z)

(aa)   (bb)

Fig. 9.4 Spermatozoa: (a) normal; (b) proximal cytoplasmic droplet (at the neck); (c) cytoplasmic droplet mid way along the mid piece; (d) distal cytoplasmic droplet (at the distal end of the mid piece); (e) and (f) oedematous acrosomes (compare with the adjacent normal sperm); (g) knobbed acrosome (upper sperm); (h) crater defect of the head, (i) undifferentiated heads; (j) abnormal attachment of the mid piece to the head (top sperm); compare with the normal sperm below; (k) broken neck; (l) detached head; (m–r) various mid piece abnormalities; (s–x) various tail abnormalities; (y) double head; (z) and (aa) double mid pieces; (bb) double mid piece and tail.

Other tests

❑   a variety of other tests are now used to assess spermatozoa, including the hypo-osmotic swelling test (a test of functional integrity of the spermatozoal membrane), and sperm penetration assays

Sample storage

❑   *always* put some of the sample into buffered formal saline (roughly 1:1), wax the bottle cap to prevent evaporation and label the bottle clearly; this provides for retrospective checking in any cases of doubt

Overall interpretation (see 15.3)

Polymorphonuclear leucocytes (neutrophils) and macrophages

❑ these may come from the prostate gland but more commonly are contaminants from the penile wall and preputial lining (see 15.2)
❑ wiping the penis to remove this film of cells before collection is resented by most dogs
❑ spermatozoa can often be seen to be adherent to macrophages, but in general the motility of the sample is not affected by polymorphonuclear leucocytes

Erythrocytes (see 6.5)

❑ these are commonly seen in the ejaculates of dogs over 5 years old
❑ they undoubtedly originate in the prostate gland, and are usually present in the absence of clinical disease
❑ even when present in large numbers, they do not appear to affect sperm motility (this is not the case in other species)

Motility

❑ may be affected by temperature and toxic substances in collection equipment
❑ in many fertile dogs 90–95% motility is seen
❑ less than 80% progressive motility may indicate a reduction in fertility

Morphology (Fig. 9.4)

❑ the staining technique may affect morphology, e.g. some preparations of nigrosin–eosin cause bending of the sperm tail
❑ the sample should be stained as soon as possible after collection
❑ less than 80% normal live spermatozoa may indicate a reduction in fertility
❑ the significance of specific sperm abnormalties is outlined below

Acrosome abnormalities

❑ the acrosome is essential for fusion of the sperm with the ovum
❑ premature lifting or separation of the acrosome may indicate early capacitation (a maturation process which usually occurs when the sperm is in the female genital tract and must occur before the sperm can penetrate an ovum)
❑ knobbed acrosomes are usually only seen in small numbers in dog semen; in other species large numbers of knobbed acrosomes cause sterility
❑ the crater defect probably indicates that parts of the DNA (genetic material) in the head have not formed properly

Neck abnormalities

❑ bending at the neck or detachment of the head may be caused by rough handling of the sample; usually very few such sperms are present in any one sample

❑ proximal cytoplasmic droplets are unilateral smooth swellings at the proximal mid piece (neck); they are remnants of the cytoplasm of the sperm precursor, the spermatid

❑ spermatozoa in the head of the epididymis normally have proximal droplets; such spermatozoa are not immediately capable of fertilization; the presence of proximal droplets probably indicates accelerated passage of spermatozoa through the epididymis

Mid piece abnormalities

❑ in some dogs infertility is caused by disruption of the continuity of the neck and mid piece associated with abnormalities of the mitochondria; irregular swellings (tags) are seen at the neck and along the rest of the mid piece

❑ distal cytoplasmic droplets are located at the distal end of the mid piece and represent migration of the proximal droplet; they are considered to be normal

Tail abnormalities

❑ abnormal shaped tails do not allow progressive movement of the sperma- tozoon and may compromise both its journey to the Fallopian tube and its ability to penetrate the ovum

Predicting fertility (see 15.3)

❑ as long as the dog has not already ejaculated on the collection day, the time of his previous ejaculation has little effect on his semen quality; however, if a dog that appears ill at case produces a sample of poor quality, a repeat examination is indicated

❑ the dog may have received drugs which will affect semen quality (see Chapter 24)

❑ as a result of semen analysis, a dog cannot be said to be fertile; fertility includes the ability to mount and copulate normally and can only be proven if the dog produces offspring

❑ dogs with seminal values described above should be fertile, i.e. if mated once or twice to bitches close to ovulation time, and should produce litters of average size for that breed from 80% or more of the bitches

❑ dogs with poor semen quality (low motility, low numbers, many abnormals) will still be fertile, but more bitches will be expected to 'miss'; repeated matings to the same bitch around her ovulation time (see 2.4) may increase the likelihood of her conceiving

❑ dogs with no spermatozoa, or very small numbers of dead, abnormal sper- matozoa, may:

(a) have been treated with anabolic steroids or other androgens; their effect is usually reversible and the ejaculate should return to normal in 2 months

(b) not have ejaculated properly, usually due to nervousness

(c) have suffered a spermatogenic arrest (see 15.3); these dogs are initially fertile but suffer a rapid, asymptomatic testicular degeneration which results in permanent aspermia

9.6   ULTRASONOGRAPHIC EXAMINATION OF THE MALE REPRODUCTIVE TRACT

Equipment for examination of the dog

❑   linear transducers are most suited to scrotal imaging, but sector transducers are adequate
❑   sector transducers are most suited to transabdominal imaging
❑   a 7.5 MHz transducer is necessary to obtain suitable image definition but a 5.0 MHz transducer offers a compromise which gives a reasonable depth of penetration combined with adequate tissue resolution
❑   the principles of ultrasonography and ultrasound terminology are given in Chapter 4

Examination of the dog

❑   cleaning of the scrotum and application of a high viscosity gel is necessary to obtain good quality images
❑   clipping the hair of the ventral abdomen is required for examination of the prostate gland
❑   in many patients imaging is most conveniently performed with the dog in the standing position

The normal testis and epididymis

❑   several imaging planes have been suggested for examination of the testes:
   (a) transverse
   (b) sagittal
   (c) dorsal
   (d) pre-scotal position (allows comparison of left and right testes)
❑   the testicular parenchyma appears relatively hypoechoic with regular diffuse echogenic stippling scattered evenly throughout the organ
❑   the stippling represents an extension of the fibrous mediastinum which is responsible for supporting the parenchymal tissue
❑   the mediastinum testis is located centrally within the tesis. In a sagittal plane this structure appears as an echogenic line approximately 2 mm wide extending from the cranial to the caudal pole, whilst in the transverse plane it appears as a central echogenic circular structure (Fig. 9.5)
❑   acoustic shadowing is often noted distal to the mediastinum testis
❑   surrounding the testis the hyperechoic summed testicular and vaginal tunics are clearly defined
❑   the head and body of the epididymis are often difficult to identify
❑   the epididymal tail has a triangular-shaped appearance
❑   the epididymis appears hypoechoic with respect to testicular parenchyma

(a)

(b)

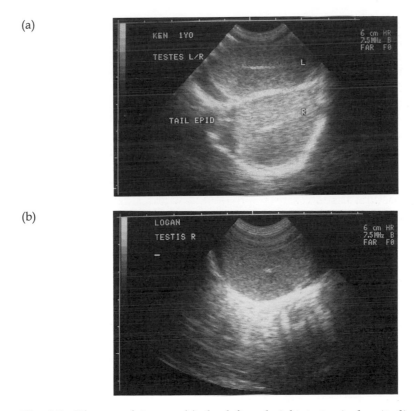

Fig. 9.5 Ultrasound image: (a) the left and right testes in longitudinal section; the hypoechoic epididymides can be clearly seen. The central echogenic line within each testis is the mediastinum testis; (b) a single testis in transverse section; the mediastinum testis appears as a central echogenic spot. 7.5 MHz transducer, scale in centimetres.

Relationship between testicular size and semen quality

❏ ultrasound can be used to accurately measure testicular size and to calculate testicular volume
❏ whilst there is a general relationship between testicular size and semen quality, this is not always the case
❏ azoospermic dogs, and dogs with severe spermatozoal abnormalities may have a normal testicular volume

The normal prostate gland

❏ examination of the prostate gland is facilitated by the presence of fluid within the bladder
❏ this can be achieved by preventing urination, or the infusion of sterile isotonic saline via a catheter
❏ imaging is achieved by placing the ultrasound transducer on the caudoventral abdomen adjacent to the prepuce

❑ imaging may be difficult if the gland lies entirely within the pelvis; however, the transducer may be placed into the dog's rectum and directed ventrally to allow adequate imaging of the caudal prostate

❑ the normal prostate gland is well circumscribed, although frequently the prostatic capsule is difficult to identify because its specular echo is sensitive to the direction of the ultrasound

❑ the gland usually has a symmetrical bilobed outline

❑ there is a midline furrow dorsal to the prostatic urethra

❑ the prostatic parenchyma is moderately echogenic, and has coarse stippling present evenly throughout the gland (Fig. 9.6)

❑ at the hilar region the prostate has linear echogenic streaks associated with peri-urethral tissue

❑ the prostatic urethra is not normally visible, although during sedation or anaesthesia this may be urine filled and appears as an anechoic line in longitudinal section

❑ in the castrated male the prostate is small and hypoechoic, the smallest size being found in dogs castrated before puberty

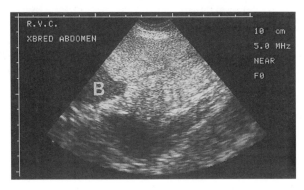

Fig. 9.6   Ultrasound image showing the bilobed prostate gland positioned at the neck of the bladder (B). 7.5 MHz transducer, scale in centimetres.

9.7   MEASUREMENT OF PLASMA HORMONES

❑ measurement of basal plasma (serum) hormone concentrations has limited application in the infertile dog

Plasma (serum) testosterone concentration

❑ testosterone concentrations vary widely throughout the day

❑ single samples are often not diagnostic

❑ basal testosterone is only useful for the demonstration of functional testicular tissue

(a) entire dogs have testosterone concentrations above 4.0 ng/ml (14.0 nmol/l)

(b) castrated dogs have testosterone concentrations below 2.0 ng/ml (7.0 nmol/l)

(c) dogs with impaired spermatogenesis have values similar to entire dogs

(d) bilaterally cryptorchid dogs have values similar to entire dogs

NB: single samples from entire dogs may be taken at the 'trough' of daily production and therefore appear basal

Plasma (serum) luteinizing hormone (LH) concentration

❏ LH is released episodically approximately every 90 minutes

❏ LH concentrations can fluctuate by up to four times basal secretion during the day

❏ increased LH concentrations may develop in cases of impaired spermatogenesis

(a) normal dogs have LH concentrations below 30 ng/ml

(b) castrated dogs have LH concentrations above 70 ng/ml

(c) dogs with impaired spermatogenesis have LH concentrations above 70 ng/ml

(d) bilaterally cryptorchid dogs have values similar to entire dogs

NB: preferably, mean values should be calculated after collecting serial samples over time

Plasma (serum) follicle-stimulating hormone (FSH) concentration

❏ FSH release fluctuates during the day but to a lesser degree than LH

❏ increased FSH concentrations may develop in cases of impaired spermatogenesis

(a) normal dogs have FSH concentrations below 70 ng/ml

(b) castrated dogs have FSH concentrations above 700 ng/ml

(c) dogs with impaired spermatogenesis have FSH concentrations above 100 ng/ml

(d) bilaterally cryptorchid dogs have values similar to entire dogs

NB: preferably, mean values should be calculated after collecting serial samples over time

9.8 OBSERVATION OF MATING BEHAVIOUR

❏ it is always important to observe mating attempts in dogs that are said to be infertile

❏ abnormalities of coitus are described in Chapter 8

9.9 BACTERIAL EXAMINATION OF THE MALE REPRODUCTIVE TRACT

❏ all male dogs have a resident commensal bacterial flora

❏ this may be associated with a persistent or recurrent mucopurulent discharge

❏ the bacteria isolated may change daily

- ❏ many species of bacteria are present, including haemolytic streptococci, staphylococci, other streptococci, *Escherichia coli*, and many others
- ❏ there is usually a mixed flora with 2–5 species present
- ❏ the incidence of anaerobic bacteria is not well documented

Interpretation of bacteriology of the prepuce

- ❏ these swabs should be expected to contain bacteria
- ❏ there is no evidence that this is a sign of clinical disease
- ❏ there is no evidence in a change in the flora following coitus
- ❏ withholding mating because of the isolation of a commensal bacterium (including β-haemolytic streptococci) seems unnecessary
- ❏ the only known bacterial venereal pathogen is *Brucella canis*
- ❏ routine bacteriological screening of the clinically normal dog is pointless

9.10 TESTICULAR BIOPSY

- ❏ biopsy allows the evaluation of spermatogenesis, and the detection of inflammatory and neoplastic cells
- ❏ biopsy is, however, very invasive and can itself cause severe testicular changes
- ❏ excisional wedge biopsy with closure of the tunica albuginea is the least traumatic method
- ❏ tissue should be fixed in Bouin's fixative and examined by an experienced histopathologist

9.11 TESTICULAR FINE NEEDLE ASPIRATION

- ❏ requires sedation preferably with a sedative/analgesic compound
- ❏ aspiration of the testicular parenchyma using a 20G needle attached to a 10 ml syringe usually gives an adequate sample
- ❏ material should be immediately fixed and stained for examination by an experienced histopathologist
- ❏ a variety of cell types including spermatocytes, spermatids and spermatozoa may be identified; Sertoli cells are easily recognized, but in normal dogs limited numbers of Leydig cells and spermatogonia are found
- ❏ subjective scoring of the percentages of each cell type may be useful when investigating infertile dogs

9.12 PROSTATIC BIOPSY

- ❏ true cut biopsies can be obtained in the anaesthetized dog using a trans-abdominal or pararectal approach
- ❏ wedge biopsy at laparotomy is the preferred method because the procedure also allows inspection of the prostate gland; this ensures that a representative sample is collected

❏ ultrasound-guided fine needle aspiration may also be useful in allowing the collection of tissue; one particular advantage is the rapid collection of material for bacteriological examination in cases of prostatic abscessation
❏ collection of the third fraction of the ejaculate should not be overlooked as a technique allowing the bacteriological and cytological evaluation of the prostate

9.13   PROSTATIC MASSAGE/URETHRAL FLUSHING

❏ prostatic fluid for bacteriological and cytological evaluation can be obtained by massage of the prostate transrectally whilst simultaneously flushing the prostatic urethra with 5–10 ml of physiological saline
❏ examination of pre- and post-massage aspirates of the urethra ensures that any cells identified originate from the prostate

9.14   ENDOCRINOLOGICAL STIMULATION TESTS

❏ measurement of basal hormone concentrations is not always diagnostic
❏ hormone stimulation tests may be useful to confirm the presence of a functional pituitary–testicular interaction (the gonadotrophin-releasing hormone (GnRH) stimulation test)
❏ hormone stimulation tests may be useful to confirm the presence of functional testicular tissue (the human chorionic gonadotrophin (hCG) stimulation test)

The gonadotrophin releasing hormone (GnRH) stimulation test

❏ a plasma (serum) sample is collected and assayed for LH and testosterone concentration
❏ a GnRH analogue is injected intravenously (0.01 µg/kg buserelin) and a second sample is assayed for LH and testosterone concentration 60 minutes later
❏ a significant increase in LH concentration indicates the presence of a functional pituitary gland
❏ a significant increase in testosterone concentration indicates the presence of a functional pituitary gland and testicle
❏ the test has not been widely evaluated and it is more common to perform an hCG stimulation test

The human chorionic gonadotrophin (hCG) stimulation test

❏ hCG is used rather than LH because the latter is not commercially available
❏ hCG is principally LH-like in activity
❏ a plasma (serum) sample is collected and assayed for testosterone concentration
❏ hCG is injected intravenously (50 IU/kg) and a second sample is assayed for testosterone concentration 60 minutes later

❏ a significant increase in testosterone concentration indicates the presence of functional testicular tissue (the test may be used to confirm the presence or absence of testicular tissue in dogs with an unknown reproductive history, e.g. apparent bilateral cryptorchidism)

9.15 KARYOTYPING

❏ may be useful in certain cases of infertility
❏ there is a limited number of institutions offering this service
❏ requires collection of blood into EDTA anticoagulant and rapid transport to the laboratory
❏ chromosomes are examined from metaphase spreads following culture

10 Fertilization

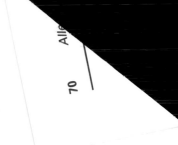

10.1 MATING TIME AND FERTILIZATION TIME

- ❏ the time of ovulation is variable in relation to the onset of pro-oestrus (Fig. 10.1)
- ❏ many breeders, however, impose standard mating regimes (usually a defined number of days after the onset of vulval bleeding) upon their animals
- ❏ bitches are often mated at an inappropriate time, and this constitutes the commonest cause of apparent infertility
- ❏ fortunately, both eggs and spermatozoa have prolonged survival in the female reproductive tract (this results in the differences between the 'apparent' and the 'actual' pregnancy length; see 11.1)

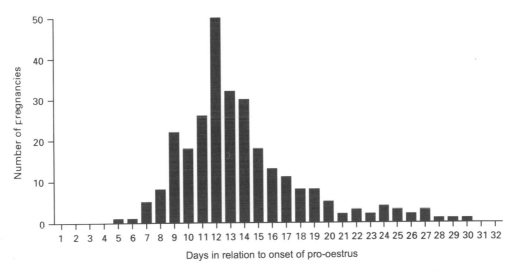

Days in relation to onset of pro-oestrus

Fig. 10.1   Relationship between day of ovulation and onset of pro-oestrus for 280 bitches.

10.2 REPRODUCTIVE PHYSIOLOGY

- ❏ the oocyte is ovulated in an immature state, and unlike other species cannot be fertilized immediately
- ❏ fertilization can only occur following maturation of the primary oocyte, extrusion of the polar body, and completion of the first meiotic division
- ❏ these events are not completed until at least 48 hours after ovulation
- ❏ ovulation occurs 2 days after the surge of plasma LH

□ oocytes remain viable within the reproductive tract for a further 4–5 days before degenerating

The 'fertilization period'

□ the time when oocytes can be fertilized
□ commences 4 days after the pre-ovulatory surge of LH
□ terminates 7 days after the pre-ovulatory surge of LH
□ therefore extends between 2 and 5 days after ovulation

The 'fertile period'

□ the time during which a mating could result in a conception
□ includes the fertilization period, but precedes it by several days, due to sperm survival within the female reproductive tract before ovulation and oocyte maturation
□ extends from 3 days before, until 7 days after, the pre-ovulatory LH surge and may be even longer for dogs with exceptional semen quality (Fig. 10.2)

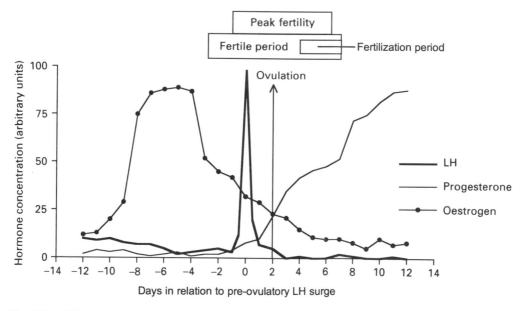

Fig. 10.2 Schematic representation of the changes in peripheral plasma hormone concentration in relation to the fertile and fertilization periods.

10.3 ASSESSING THE OPTIMAL TIME FOR MATING

□ likely to be during, or immediately preceding the fertilization period
□ the period of peak fertility for natural matings ranges from 1 day before, until 6 days after, the LH surge

❏   determination of the optimal time to mate can be assessed by measuring the LH surge, or by methods that reliably indicate the fertile or preferably the fertilization period

❏   when the use of preserved semen is contemplated, insemination should be performed only during the fertilization period, to ensure success

Clinical assessments

Counting the number of days

❏   many dogs breeders rely upon counting the number of days from the onset of pro-oestrus

❏   many dog breeders believe that bitches always ovulate a defined number of days from the onset of this pro-oestrus; *this is not true*

❏   while the 'average bitch' may ovulate 12 days after the onset of pro-oestrus
    (a) some bitches ovulate as early as day 5 after the onset of pro-oestrus
    (b) some bitches ovulate as late as day 30 after the onset of pro-oestrus (Fig. 10.1)

❏   mating on the 12th and 14th days, which is common breeding practice, may therefore fail to result in conception

Oestrous behaviour

❏   initial studies suggested that the onset of standing oestrus occurred at the same time as the LH surge

❏   using these data, mating 4 days after the onset of standing oestrus would be a suitable time

❏   however, in many bitches the behavioural events have been shown to correlate poorly with the underlying hormonal events

Vulval softening

❏   during pro-oestrus the vulva and perineal tissues become enlarged, oedematous and somewhat turgid

❏   distinct vulval softening often occurs at the time of the LH surge

❏   this is related to a change from high oestrogen concentration to low oestrogen concentration with rising progesterone

❏   mating should commence 4 days after the onset of vulval softening

❏   when clinical assessments alone are available, the combination of the onset of standing oestrus and the timing of vulval softening may be useful because each event occurs, on average, 4 days before the beginning of the fertilization period

Measurement of plasma hormones (see 4.9)

❏   measurement of the plasma concentration of LH is a reliable and accurate method for determining the optimum time to mate

❏   but there is no readily available commercial assay for canine LH

❏ however, in the bitch, plasma progesterone concentration begins to increase from baseline approximately 2 days before ovulation (the result of pre-ovulatory luteinization)

❏ serial monitoring of plasma progesterone therefore allows:
   (a) anticipation of ovulation
   (b) confirmation of ovulation
   (c) detection of the fertilization period

❏ the initial rise in progesterone is gradual; therefore it is only necessary to collect blood samples every second or third day

❏ mating or insemination should be planned between 4 and 6 days after the plasma progesterone concentration exceeds 2.0 ng/ml (6.5 nmol/l) (the value at the time of the LH surge), or should preferably commence 1 day after values exceed 8–10.0 ng/ml (25.0–32.0 nmol/l) (the beginning of the fertilization period)

❏ progesterone may be measured by radioimmunoassay or an enzyme-linked immunosorbent assay (ELISA) test kit (see 4.9)

Vaginal cytology (see 4.5)

❏ collection, staining and microscopic examination of exfoliated vaginal cells is a simple method for monitoring the stage of the oestrous cycle

❏ the relative proportions of different types of epithelial cell can be used as markers of the endocrine environment

❏ the fertile (not fertilization) period can be predicted by calculating the percentage of epithelial cells that appear anuclear when using a modified Wright–Giemsa stain

❏ mating should be attempted throughout the period when:
   (a) more than 80% of epithelial cells are anuclear (the fertile period) (Fig. 10.3)
   (b) polymorphonuclear leucocytes are absent from the smear

❏ at the end of the fertilization period, plasma progesterone concentrations remain high and there is sloughing of much of the vaginal epithelium

❏ the termination of the fertile period can be detected when:
   (a) the percentage of large irregularly-shaped anuclear cells decreases
   (b) polymorphonuclear leucocytes reappear in large numbers
   (c) the vaginal smear is dominated by small epithelial cells, cellular debris, and bacteria

❏ whilst vaginal cytology is a useful technique it should be remembered that:
   (a) polymorphonuclear leucocytes may be found throughout the fertile period in some bitches
   (b) in some bitches peak values of only 60% anuclear cells are reached

Vaginal endoscopy

❏ vaginoscopic assessment is based upon observation of:
   (a) mucosal fold contours and profiles

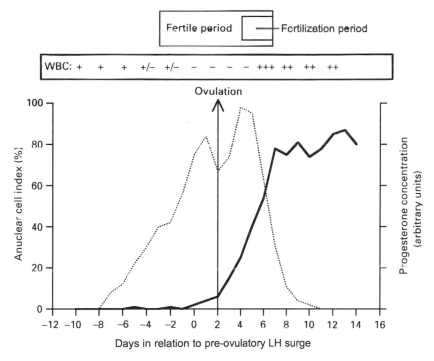

Fig. 10.3 Schematic representation of the changes in the anuclear cell index (dotted line), plasma progesterone concentration (solid line) and number of polymorphonuclear leucocytes (WBC) in relation to the fertile and fertilization periods.

   (b) the colour of the mucosa

   (c) the colour of any fluid present

❑ at the onset of pro-oestrus and during early oestrus the mucosal folds are enlarged, oedematous, and pink or pink/white in colour

❑ these changes are due to thickening of the mucosal epithelium, and oedema accumulation within the submucosa

❑ at the time of the LH surge there is progressive shrinking of the folds accompanied by pallor

❑ subsequently, mucosal shrinkage is accompanied by wrinkling of the mucosal folds which become distinctly angulated and a dense-cream to white colour

❑ the onset of the fertile period can be detected by observing mucosal shrinkage without angulation

❑ shrinkage with angulation is characteristic of the fertilization period

❑ mating or insemination should be planned during the fertilization period, or 4–6 days after first detecting mucosal shrinkage

❑ the termination of the fertilization period can be detected by observing a decline or cessation of mucosal shrinkage, combined with sloughing of the vaginal epithelium

Examination of cervico-vaginal secretion

❏ the electrical resistance of the vaginal secretions decreases during late oestrus, but the technique has been poorly investigated in the domestic bitch
❏ some workers claim that the concentration of glucose within the vaginal discharge can be used to predict the optimal mating time, but the technique has failed to stand up to scientific investigation
❏ crystallization of mucus collected from the anterior vagina may be useful in combination with vaginal cytology for determining the optimal mating time (see 4.5)

11 Pregnancy

depends on how it is calculated:

from 1st mating: 58-72 days
from LH peak: 64-66 days
from Day 1: 56-59 days
P4 levels generally low but don't count on it.

11.1 PREGNANCY LENGTH

❑ this is usually taken to be the interval between the first mating and parturition

❑ on this basis, <u>pregnancy length may vary between 58 and 72 days</u>; this is termed the apparent pregnancy length   *58-72 days*

❑ fertile matings have been recorded between 9 days before and 5 days after ovulation

❑ the interval between the luteinizing hormone peak (see 3.3) and the day of parturition is consistently 64–66 days; this is termed the actual pregnancy length

❑ <u>the expected day of parturition can be predicted in the bitch by measurement of the decline in plasma progesterone concentration which occurs 24–36</u> hours earlier. Progesterone can be easily measured using an ELISA technique in the practice laboratory

❑ coincidental with the decline in progesterone is a decrease in rectal temperature. This pre-partum hypothermia may be detected clinically and be useful for predicting parturition

❑ on average bitches whelp 57 days after the onset of cytological metoestrus (see 2.5 and 4.5)   *LH → preg 64-66 days*

11.2 ENDOCRINE CHANGES IN BLOOD (Fig. 3.1)

Progesterone *– CL sole site of production*

❑ concentrations of progesterone are similar during pregnancy to those in metoestrus (see 3.5)

❑ the uterus does not synthesize progesterone as in other species and the <u>corpora lutea are the sole site</u> of production

❑ in late pregnancy progesterone concentrations are relatively low, but fall sharply when the corpora lutea are lysed 24–36 hours pre-partum

Oestrogen

❑ concentrations are probably the same in pregnancy as metoestrus; reported differences may reflect measurement of different oestrogens by different assay systems

❑ <u>oestrogen concentrations increase steadily throughout pregnancy and reach peak values immediately before parturition</u>

❑ concentrations decrease abruptly to basal after parturition

Prolactin

❑ concentrations increase in the latter half of pregnancy, as progesterone concentrations decrease
❑ similar changes occur in non-pregnant bitches and are associated with false pregnancy (see 2.7), although the broad rise in prolactin during the second half of pregnancy appears to be clearly greater than most non-pregnant cycles
❑ there is a transient large surge during the decline in progesterone 24–36 hours before parturition
❑ prolactin concentrations are elevated but fluctuate during lactation

Relaxin

❑ concentrations start to increase from the 25th day; this can be used as a pregnancy test
❑ peak values occur at days 40–50 and are followed by a slight decline before parturition
❑ relaxin is the only known pregnancy-specific hormone in the dog

11.3 DEVELOPMENT OF THE CONCEPTUS

❑ eggs are ovulated as *primary oocytes*
❑ oocyte maturation to produce the *secondary oocyte* with extrusion of the polar body occurs during the 3 days after ovulation
❑ the secondary oocyte (*ovum*) can be fertilized from 3 days until about 5 days after ovulation
❑ fertilization occurs in the distal Fallopian (uterine) tube
❑ the fertilized ovum is called the *zygote*
❑ rapid division (cleavage) of the zygote produces a *morula* which is a solid ball of cells
❑ the morulae enter the uterus from the Fallopian tubes at about 9 days after ovulation, i.e. about 6 days after fertilization
❑ a cavity (the *blastocoele*) develops rapidly in the centre of the morula (which is now composed of about 30 cells) and the resulting fluid-filled sphere is called a *blastocyst*
❑ the single-cell-thick wall of the blastocyst will develop into the fetal membranes which contribute to the placenta; a small button of cells to one side of the cavity, the inner cell mass, will mainly give rise to the *embryo* proper
❑ until this stage the developing embryo has remained the same size as the original ovum because it has been surrounded by a non-cellular membrane, the *zona pellucida*; with successive divisions the cells have become smaller
❑ disappearance of the zona pellucida allows the developing conceptus to increase in size
❑ the conceptuses grow and arrange themselves in a roughly even manner along the uterine horns, but are not attached to the endometrium until 21 days after ovulation

❏ between the 21st and 40th day, each growing conceptus is roughly spherical
❏ until the 35th day, there is a portion of constricted uterus between each of these discrete conceptuses (Fig. 11.1)
❏ after 35 days, continued growth of the conceptuses expands the constrictions, so that adjacent chorio-allantoic membranes come into contact with each other and both uterine horns become uniformally distended
❏ early in pregnancy there is a relatively large amount of fetal fluid (mainly in the yolk sac) compared with the size of the developing puppy (embryo)
❏ at about 35 days the arrangement of cells within the embryo, i.e. the process of *organogenesis*, is complete and thereafter the developing individual is called a *fetus*; its subsequent development is mainly due to an increase in size
❏ as pregnancy develops, the allantois becomes the main fluid-filled cavity in the conceptus, but the volume of fluid becomes relatively reduced compared

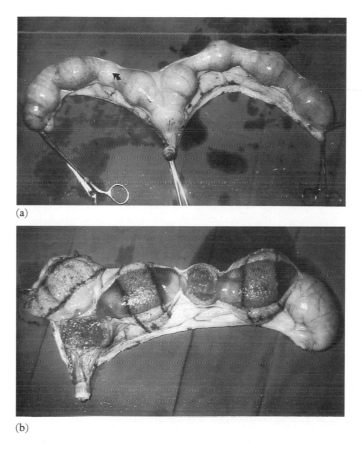

(a)

(b)

Fig. 11.1 Uterus in mid pregnancy: (a) immediately after ovariohysterectomy; note the small conceptual swelling (arrowed); (b) partial dissection of the uterus; resorption sites can be seen in the body and right horn (shown on the left in a). The zonary nature of the placenta and the marginal haematoma are clearly illustrated.

with the size of the growing fetus; in the early stages the very delicate embryo requires cushioning (by fluid) from external stimuli; the larger fetus is more robust and needs less 'protection'
❏ the small amount of fetal fluid that remains at parturition acts as a lubricant during birth

11.4 DEVELOPMENT OF THE PLACENTA

❏ at around the 21st day after ovulation, a permanent attachment begins to develop between each conceptus and the endometrium; this process in the bitch is best described as *nidation* (and sometimes wrongly called implantation) and results in the formation of the *placenta*
❏ the *placenta* is the union between the outer set of fetal membranes (the *allantochorion*) and the lining of the uterus (the endometrium)
❏ very vascular finger-like *villi* on the surface of the allantochorion fit tightly into cavities (*crypts*) in the endometrium; exchange of gases and nutrients occurs between the circulatory systems (capillaries) of the dam and fetus in the placentae
❏ the placenta of the dog is described as being *zonary*, i.e. there is a band of placental attachment around the centre of each conceptus (Fig. 11.1)
❏ over most of this placental area the epithelium and connective tissue of the endometrium are lost, so that the villi are in direct contact with maternal capillaries; the placenta is said to be *endotheliochorial*
❏ along both edges of the placental zone the maternal blood vessels rupture; the leaked blood is contained along the periphery of the placenta and is called the haemochorial border or *marginal haematoma*
❏ the marginal haematomas contain large pools of stagnant maternal blood from which the extra-embryonic circulation absorbs various metabolites, especially iron
❏ destruction of the blood pigment haemoglobin in this marginal haematoma produces the green *uteroverdin*; this is seen when placentae start to break down at parturition

11.5 OTHER CHANGES DURING PREGNANCY

Abdominal enlargement

❏ in pregnancy this is not noticeable until 45–50 days
❏ overfeeding may mimic pregnancy
❏ the total bodyweight of the bitch may increase 20–55% during gestation

Mammary development

❏ an increase in blood supply may be seen in all bitches, around 25–30 days after ovulation, i.e. the veins around the base of the nipples become more prominent

❑ continued development to produce milk occurs in both pregnancy and pseudopregnancy (see 2.7)

Blood changes

❑ at about 33–37 days of gestation there is an increase in concentrations of acute phase proteins in blood; this is being used as a method of pregnancy diagnosis (see 12.8)
❑ a progressive anaemia starts during the third week of pregnancy; it appears not to affect the health of the bitch:
   (a) the packed cell volume (PCV) is usually less than 40% at day 35 and below 35% at term
   (b) the major cause of the anaemia is the result of increased plasma volume causing haemodilution
❑ sensitivity to insulin, but not glucagon, is reduced and this may aggravate pre-existing diabetes mellitus

Appetite

❑ this is usually depressed during mid pregnancy; it does not affect the growth of pups but may alarm the owner
❑ the requirement for available carbohydrate is increased in later pregnancy and appetite then increases
❑ during late pregnancy the bitch should be given several small meals a day

Mucoid vulval discharge

❑ this is often present, and must be distinguished from the pathological discharge due to pyometra, which occurs at the same stage of the cycle (see 14.5)

12 Pregnancy Diagnosis

In most domestic species pregnancy interrupts normal cyclical activity by increasing the length of the luteal phase and delaying the return to oestrus. The physiology of the bitch is unlike other species in that the luteal phase is similar in length for both pregnancy and non-pregnancy. In addition, the fertilization period of the bitch differs from most other mammals. In particular it should be remembered that:

❑ in most bitches the day of ovulation is not known and both 'early' and 'late' matings can result in a pregnancy:
(a) matings that occur before ovulation may be fertile should spermatozoa reside within the reproductive tract 'waiting' for ovulation; an 'early' mating produces an apparently long pregnancy length
(b) oocytes may then remain fertilizable for at least 5 days after ovulation; a 'late' mating produces an apparently short pregnancy length
(c) bitches may be examined soon after mating for pregnancy diagnosis; if the mating was 'early' this may result in a false negative diagnosis, because the examination was undertaken before a positive diagnosis could be made
❑ endocrinological methods of pregnancy diagnosis cannot simply be adapted from other species

12.1 ABSENCE OF A RETURN TO OESTRUS

[handwritten margin note: cannot be used as means of preg. detection in the bitch]

❑ in the bitch the inter-oestrous interval is identical in pregnant and non-pregnant cycles
❑ an absence of a return to oestrus is not specific for pregnancy

12.2 BEHAVIOURAL CHANGES *– limited use*

❑ both pregnant and non-pregnant bitches may exhibit behavioural changes typical of pregnancy
❑ these are usually associated with an increase in plasma prolactin concentration
❑ food intake may increase in both pregnant and non-pregnant bitches

12.3 PHYSICAL CHANGES

❑ pregnant bitches commonly have a small volume mucoid vulval discharge approximately 1 month after mating
❑ body weight begins to increase from day 35 of pregnancy

❑ abdominal swelling may be noted from day 40 of pregnancy
☑ mammary gland enlargement is usually obvious from day 35, at which time serous fluid can be expressed from the glands
❑ colostrum may be present in the teats in the last 7 days of pregnancy
NB: similar features are common in pseudopregnant bitches

12.4 ABDOMINAL PALPATION

❑ can be highly accurate
❑ may be difficult in obese or nervous animals
❑ may be inaccurate if the bitch was mated 'early' such that pregnancy is not as advanced as anticipated

– not accurate for puppy count

Technique

Small dogs

❑ one hand can be used for abdominal palpation
❑ abdominal contents are then allowed to pass between the fingers and thumb as the hand is drawn ventrally

Large dogs

❑ a two handed technique is preferable
❑ ideally the owner and clinician should be seated and facing each other
❑ the owner holds the bitch's head
❑ then the clinician's extended hands are placed on either side of the abdomen, mid way between the anterior pelvis and last rib
❑ both hands simultaneously compress the abdomen and are then moved dorsally so that viscera slip between the fingers

Interpretation

❑ the optimum time for diagnosis is approximately 1 month after mating
(a) the conceptuses are spherical in outline, and may vary between 15 and 30 mm in diameter
(b) they are tense fluid-filled structures and can be readily palpated
❑ from day 35 the conceptuses become elongated, enlarged and tend to lose their tenseness; they may be less easy to palpate at this time
❑ after day 45 the uterine horns tend to fold upon themselves, resulting in the caudal portion of each horn being positioned against the ventral abdominal wall, and the cranial portion of the same horn being positioned dorsally
❑ after day 55 the fetuses can often be identified, especially if the forequarters of the bitch are elevated and the uterus is manipulated caudally towards the pelvis
❑ it is difficult to accurately count the number of conceptuses by palpation except when performing an early examination

12.5 IDENTIFICATION OF FETAL HEART BEATS

- ❏ in late pregnancy it is possible to auscultate fetal heart beats using a stethoscope
- ❏ fetal hearts may also be detected by recording a fetal electrocardiogram (ECG) – *difficult unless & quiet*
- ❏ both methods are diagnostic of pregnancy
- ❏ fetal heart beats are simple to detect because the heart rate is usually more than twice that of the dam

✓ *U/s useful*

12.6 RADIOGRAPHY

- ❏ uterine enlargement can be detected from day 30
- ❏ at this stage the enlarged uterus can be readily identified in the caudal abdomen, originating dorsal to the bladder and ventral to the rectum; it frequently produces cranial displacement of the small intestine
- ❏ the early pregnant uterus has only soft tissue opacity and cannot be differentiated from other causes of uterine enlargement, such as pyometra
- ❏ correct pregnancy diagnosis is not possible until after day 45 when mineralization of the fetal skeleton is detectable
- ❏ progressive mineralization results in an increasing number of bones that can be identified (Fig. 12.1) *← starts proximally*
- ❏ it is unlikely that the fetuses will be damaged by the ionizing radiation after day 45; however,
  (a) earlier examination during organogenesis is potentially hazardous
  (b) sedation or anaesthesia of the dam may be required and is a potential risk
- ❏ in late pregnancy the number of pups can be reliably estimated by counting the number of fetal skulls

12.7 ENDOCRINOLOGICAL TESTS

- ❏ plasma (serum) concentrations of progesterone are *not* useful for the diagnosis of pregnancy
- ❏ pregnancy-specific changes in plasma and urine oestrogen concentration have *not* been adequately evaluated
- ❏ a significant elevation of plasma prolactin occurs in pregnant bitches compared with non-pregnant bitches but this method has *not* been adequately evaluated   *cats ↑se CL earlier in cases of pseudopregnancy*
- ❏ measurement of the hormone relaxin *is* diagnostic of pregnancy; however, at present there is no available commercial assay for relaxin

12.8 ACUTE PHASE PROTEINS

- ❏ an acute phase response occurs in pregnant bitches at approximately the time of implantation

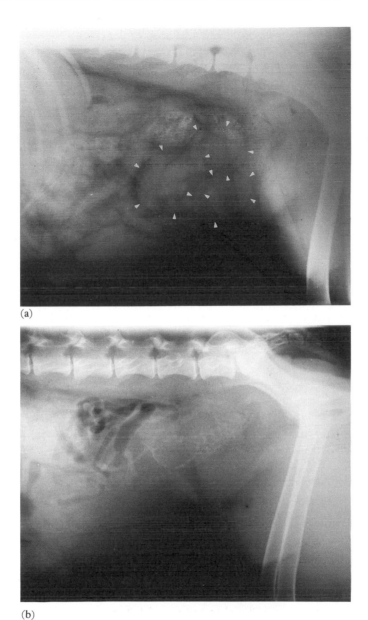

Rads-
uterine
enlargement
can be detected
@ day 30.

(a)

(b)

Fig. 12.1 Radiographs of pregnancy: (a) 28 days after mating; shadows of spherical conceptuses are delineated by the arrows and the colon is displaced dorsally. A similar picture may be seen in pyometra, see Fig. 14.5, pp. 104–105; (b) 24 hours after the apparent completion of whelping; a single pup with a flexed spine is present.

❏ this response appears to be unique to the bitch
❏ measurement of fibrinogen, C-reactive protein, or other acute phase proteins are all sensitive markers of pregnancy
  the initial rise in these proteins occurs from day 20 onwards with a peak at approximately day 40
  false positive diagnoses may result from inflammatory conditions (such as pyometra which occurs at the same stage of the oestrous cycle)
  the rise in fibrinogen concentration is now the basis of a commercial pregnancy test

12.9 ULTRASOUND EXAMINATION (see also 4.8)

Early pregnancy (Fig. 12.2)

❏ conceptuses may be first imaged from 15 days after ovulation
   (a) they appear as spherical anechoic structures approximately 2 mm in diameter. The anechoic fluid is the yolk sac, and it is not until the yolk sac is filled with a sufficient volume of fluid that the pregnancy can first be imaged
   (b) Uterine enlargement occurs during the luteal phase whether the bitch is pregnant or non-pregnant and is not specific for pregnancy
❏ during early pregnancy the embryo is located adjacent to the uterine wall and is not imaged
❏ the conceptus rapidly increases in size and may lose its spherical outline, becoming oblate in appearance
❏ from day 20 after ovulation the conceptus is approximately 7 mm in diameter and 15 mm in length, and the embryo can be imaged
❏ the presence of the embryonic heart beat can be detected from approximately 22 days after ovulation
❏ the developing allantois initially appears as a nearly spherical structure within the conceptus which subsequently increases in size and surrounds the yolk sac

(a)

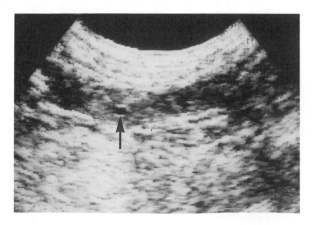

Fig. 12.2

(b)

(c)

(d)

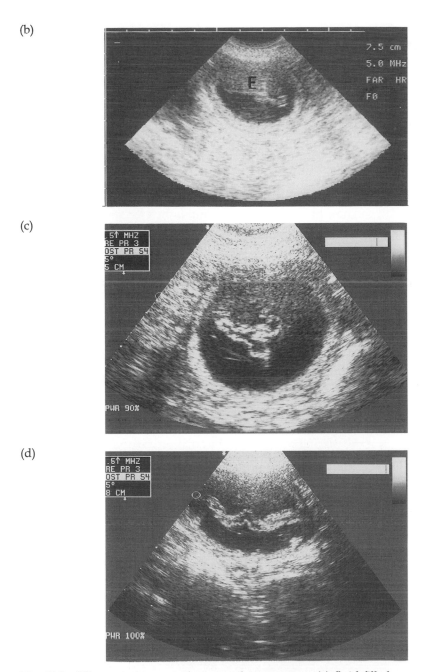

Fig. 12.2 Ultrasound images during early pregnancy: (a) fluid-filled conceptus (arrow) within one uterine horn 21 days after ovulation; (b) larger fluid-filled conceptus containing an embryo (E) and developing embryonic membranes; (c) conceptus 30 days after ovulation, demonstrating the corrugated appearance of the collapsing yolk sac in transverse section; (d) the same conceptus at 30 days after ovulation, demonstrating the yolk sac in longitudinal section. 7.5 MHz transducer, scale in centimetres.

❏ a third fluid filled sac, the amnion, may be noted later in pregnancy since it surrounds, and initially is in close apposition to, the fetus

Mid pregnancy (Fig. 12.3)

☒ the most rapid growth of the fetus occurs between days 32 and 55; during this time the limb buds become apparent and there is clear differentiation of the head, trunk and abdomen
❏ the zonary placenta can usually be easily identified from this stage of pregnancy onwards
❏ the fetal skeleton becomes evident from day 40 onwards when fetal bone appears hyperechoic, and casts acoustical shadows
❏ the heart can now be easily identified and large arteries and veins can be seen cranially and caudally
❏ lung tissue surrounding the heart is hyperechoic with respect to the liver

(a)

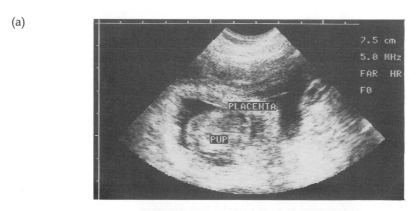

(b)

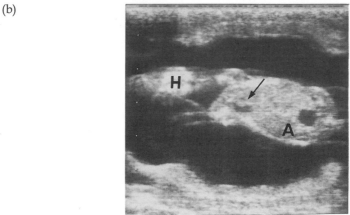

Fig. 12.3 Ultrasound images during mid pregnancy: (a) a single fetus surrounded by a small volume of fluid imaged in transverse section; (b) a single fetus imaged in longitudinal section demonstrating the fetal head (H), thorax containing the heart (arrow), and abdomen (A) containing the anechoic bladder. 5.0 MHz transducer, scale in centimetres.

❑ from 45 days onwards it is possible to identify the fluid-filled (anechoic) stomach, and a few days later the bladder can be imaged

Hydraminion will result if fetus is alive but cannot swallow

Late pregnancy (Fig. 12.4)

❑ the head, spinal column and ribs produce intense reflections and are easily identifiable
❑ in the last 20 days of gestation the kidneys can be seen
❑ the small intestine may be detected
❑ at this stage the fetus is highly mobile, and limb and whole body movements occur frequently
❑ swallowing movements can be observed
❑ hiccuping may occasionally be noticed
❑ it is difficult to examine more than a few fetuses at this time without clipping an excessive amount of hair

U/S useful to evaluate : puppy viability, placental abnormalities

Assessment of fetal number

difficult to do puppy counts due to 1g. fetuse

❑ the accuracy of detecting absolute fetal number is poor
☒ the greatest accuracy is at the first examination 1 month after mating (30d)
❑ the lowest accuracy is in late pregnancy
❑ most commonly the number of fetuses is underestimated
☒ the accuracy is reduced in large litters

Errors with real-time ultrasonography

small litters +/- 1 puppy
large litters +/- 2 puppies
missing more common than overestimating

False positive

❑ such scans are unlikely; the urinary bladder is the only viscus likely to be confused with the uterus
❑ resorption of several conceptuses has been seen and may account for the absence of puppies after a positive scan

False negative

❑ failure to detect early pregnancies may occur because:
   (a) the pregnancy may be less than 23 days
   (b) in small litters the conceptuses may be obscured by intestine (gas)

Overestimation of fetal numbers

❑ this may occur because of:
   (a) subsequent resorption
   (b) counting the same conceptus twice

Underestimation of fetal numbers

❑ this is very likely, particularly in litters of greater than four

(a)   (b)

(c)   (d)

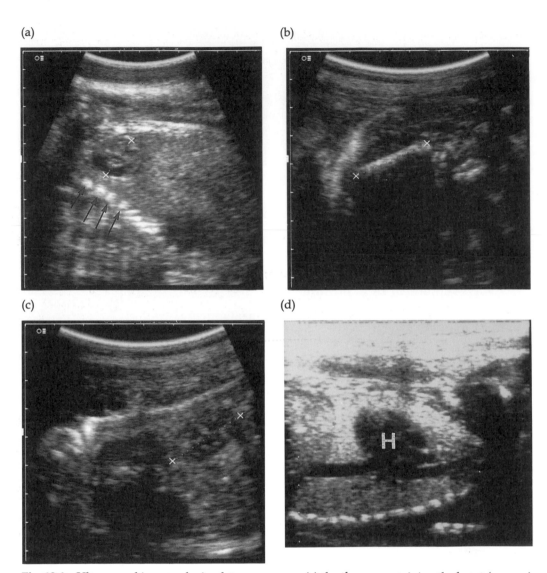

Fig. 12.4 Ultrasound images during late pregnancy: (a) the thorax containing the heart (crosses) surrounded by the lungs; the ribs are clearly visible (arrows); (b) a fetal femur (arrows) with distal acoustic shadowing; (c) a fetal kidney (crosses); (d) the fetal heart (H) with great vessels, surrounding lung, liver and diaphragm clearly visible. 5.0 MHz transducer, scale in centimetres.

Full term dead fetuses

❏ these can be overlooked because there are few obvious features; fetal ribs are most likely to be seen

13 Normal Parturition

13.1 ENDOCRINE CONTROL

❏ parturition is usually protracted in the bitch and its endocrine control is poorly understood
❏ the major endocrine event is a rapid and large increase in the oestrogen: progesterone ratio
❏ progesterone concentrations are decreasing throughout the latter part of pregnancy but fall precipitously 24–36 hours before parturition; this coincides with a fall in body temperature (see 13.3)
❏ maternal cortisol concentrations rise just before parturition but their role is not fully understood
❏ oestrogens, oxytocin and relaxin are probably involved in the initiation of parturition, as may be prostaglandins which increase in blood 36 hours pre-partum and probably cause luteolysis
❏ prolactin concentrations rise during the latter part of pregnancy and peak during lactation; prolactin is probably not involved in the initiation of parturition
❏ the trigger for the timing of parturition is likely to involve the maturation of the fetal pituitary–adrenal axis at the completion of fetal development

13.2 PREPARATION OF THE ENVIRONMENT

❏ there is no single perfect whelping area/box but the following should be considered

Draught

❏ absence of draught is important

Temperature

❏ artificial heat may be provided, but the bitch should be a good source of warmth
❏ initially a temperature of about 26°C is ideal, but if overhead heating is supplied, ensure that the bitch cannot burn (she will be closer to the lamp than the pups)

Bedding

❏ provision of material which is easily removed and disposed of when soiled

❏ a thick bed of newspaper is ideal as the top layers can be removed as necessary

Quietness

❏ the whelping box should be in the corner of a room or, better still, in a separate room
❏ this prevents the bitch from being unwittingly disturbed during whelping
❏ do not invite the neighbours in to watch

Bitch's movement

❏ provision for the bitch to be able to get away from the pups when they are older

13.3 PREPARATION OF THE BITCH

Before mating

Vaccination

❏ ensure vaccination status is up to date
❏ this means that there are adequate antibodies present in the bitch's colostrum

Other treatment

❏ any other disease of a possibly infectious nature should be treated
❏ the bitch should be wormed (prolonged courses of the newer anthelminitics, Fenbendazole and Oxfendazole, in later pregnancy will kill migrating larvae)
❏ ensure that any gingivitis is treated (by descaling teeth if necessary)
❏ drug administration should, however, be avoided during organogenesis if possible

Late pregnancy

❏ check for fleas and ear mites
❏ do not force extra food on the bitch; it is rarely necessary to increase the volume of food before about 40 days of gestation
❏ feed small amounts and often
❏ avoid calcium supplementation; this may depress parathyroid function and prevent mobilization of calcium at parturition leading to inertia (see 20.1) or eclampsia (see 20.15)
❏ introduce the bitch to the whelping area at least 2 weeks before expected parturition and get her used to sleeping there
❏ monitor mammary development in the last week; if this appears inadequate, or if nipple numbers are low compared with the expected size of the litter, have milk supplements on hand

❑ in long haired breeds it is advisable to cut hair away from the mammary glands to make the nipples more accessible and from the perineum and back legs to make cleaning the bitch easier after whelping

Temperature monitoring (Fig. 13.1)

❑ start taking the bitch's rectal temperature about 1 week before the expected whelping date
❑ temperature should be taken *at least* three times a day
❑ normal temperature is about 38°C (100.5°F) during late pregnancy
❑ a fall below 37.5°C (99.5°F) indicates that paturition should start within 24 hours (Fig. 13.1)
❑ the temperature drop may only be transient, but if temperature is taken three times daily, a single low reading may be due to incorrect procedure
❑ if no signs of whelping occur within 48 hours after the temperature fall, the bitch may be suffering from primary uterine inertia (see 20.1) and may require a caesarean operation
❑ temperature monitoring is essential in bitches known to be carrying small (one or two pups) or large litters, as these are most prone to inertia

13.4 THE 'OVERDUE' BITCH

❑ pregnancy length is remarkably consistent at 64–66 days from the LH peak (see 3.3)

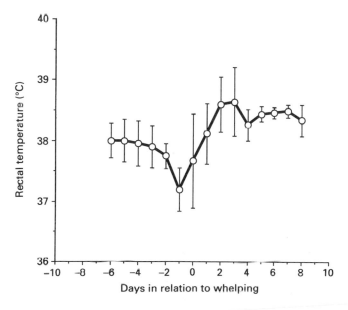

Fig. 13.1 Mean rectal temperature for five periparturient bitches.

❏ however, when measured from first or last matings, pregnancy lengths can be very variable
❏ longer than expected pregnancies can be due to:
(a) bitch being mated several days after ovulation; she can still become pregnant
(b) bitch not being pregnant! – this can be investigated by radiographic or ultrasound examination (see 12.6 and 12.9)
(c) mating dates being incorrect
(d) pregnancy length being miscalculated
(e) primary uterine inertia (see 20.1)

13.5 FIRST STAGE PARTURITION

❏ For 2–3 days before parturition bitches are often restless, seek seclusion, and eat less food possibly in response to elevated prolactin concentrations
❏ the beginning of first stage cannot be accurately recognized
❏ this is the preparation for the expulsive (second) stage
❏ there is usually milk in the mammary glands
❏ uterine contractions initially are not very frequent and the cervix is closed; some bitches are more upset by these contractions than others
❏ the onset of uterine contractions is closely related to the fall in circulating progesterone concentrations
❏ gradually the contractions appear to become more intense and frequent as a pup is being pushed towards the dilating cervix
❏ the time at which the cervix dilates fully cannot be ascertained because the bitch's vagina is relatively long and the cervix is unlikely to be reached by digital examination
❏ accurate examination of cervical patency requires endoscopic examination
❏ the allantochorion of the first pup ruptures in the vagina; the presence of a pup and its fluid and membranes in the vagina usually stimulates abdominal straining, although some pups are born with very little evidence of this
❏ the beginning of straining, or the appearance of fetal fluid or a pup at the vulva, marks the change from first to second stage parturition
❏ uterine contractions during first stage parturition may cause:
(a) restlessness
(b) anorexia
(c) panting and a 'worried look'
(d) shivering
(e) nesting behaviour
(f) looking at the flanks
(g) vulval licking
(h) vomiting if recently fed
(i) swelling and relaxation of the vulva
(j) appearance of mucus at the vulva
(k) abdominal relaxation which allows easier palpation of the fetuses

NB: the length (0–36 hours), intensity and behavioural characteristics are very variable, even in successive pregnancies in the same bitch

13.6 SECOND STAGE PARTURITION

❏ usually the amnion (water bag) of the first pup is seen at the vulva soon after straining begins
❏ passage of the head through the vulva may cause signs of pain in primigravida, but the pup is usually born with little effort
❏ pups can only be born normally in longitudinal presentation, i.e. the long axis of the puppy is parallel to the long axis of the bitch (see 20.5)
❏ anterior presentation (with the pup's head born first) is most common, but posterior presentations occur so frequently as to be accepted as normal; however, obstructive dystocia may be caused by posterior presentation of the first pup
❏ the position of the pup during normal birth is dorsal, i.e. the back of the pup is uppermost, towards the back of the dam; this allows the natural curve of the pup's spine to correspond with the curved course it must take – initially upwards into the bitch's pelvis then downwards through the vulva (Fig. 13.2)
❏ the posture of the pup is a description of the disposition of its head and legs; the legs may be either extended or flexed during normal parturition, but in anterior presentation the head and neck must be extended, i.e. the nose is leading, or obstruction will occur
❏ a breach birth is a posterior presentation with the hind limbs flexed, i.e. the feet are extended forward and the tail is seen first
❏ after the birth of the pup the bitch will lick and rupture the amnion, and rupture the umbilical cord; further licking helps to dry and stimulate the pup
NB: it is important to ensure that excess nibbling, especially at the umbilicus, does not occur; this may result in an umbilical hernia or the bitch eating part of the pup
❏ the allantochorion (see 11.4) (placenta or afterbirth) may be expelled at a variable time after the pup, and some pups are born within it; a second pup may follow before the expulsion of the first allantochorion
❏ the bitch will usually attempt to eat the allantochorion; it is not necessary that she does so and it will probably cause her to develop diarrhoea
❏ the interval between the delivery of successive pups is very variable
❏ delivery from each horn is usually alternate
❏ it is often difficult to decide when a problem has arisen; as a rough guide unproductive straining for 30 minutes may indicate an obstruction, although a normal pup may be born after this time
❏ if more pups are expected and the bitch is restless, will not let the pups suck for long, but is not straining, 2–3 hours may elapse without trouble ensuing
❏ longer periods (up to 6 hours) may occur between successive pups with the bitch showing no signs of discomfort

(a)

(b)

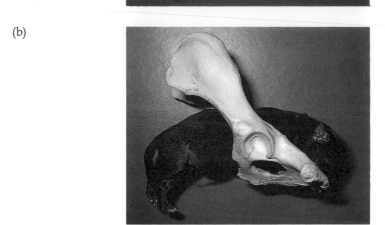

Fig. 13.2   (a, b) Normal presentation, position and posture in the dog fetus. The most common orientation is anterior longitudinal presentation, in dorsal position with the head and limbs extended rostrally. The pups move upwards to the pelvic inlet and then downwards through the vagina, vestibule and vulva.

13.7 THIRD STAGE PARTURITION

❑ classically, third stage parturition is the passage of the allantochorion
❑ in the bitch this process occurs throughout the second stage and cannot be simply defined
❑ however, involution of the empty uterus could be said to constitute a third stage, although its duration would be hard to define

13.8 INDUCTION OF PARTURITION

❑ this is not successful in the bitch
❑ administration of corticosteroids has been said to initiate parturition, but since they are given at a time when whelping is expected anyway, assessment of results is difficult

❏ oxytocin may stimulate uterine contractions in cases of primary uterine inertia if it is felt sure that the cervix has relaxed; this can only be evaluated adequately by endoscopic examination

14 Abnormalities of the Reproductive Tract of the Bitch

14.1 VULVA

Stenosis of the vulval opening

❏ this is rare; surgical correction is not difficult (see 27.7)

Perivulval dermatitis (Fig. 14.1)

❏ this is relatively common in entire bitches and those that have been neutered either before or after the first oestrus
❏ sometimes incorrectly referred to as 'juvenile vulva' or 'vulval hypoplasia'; close inspection shows the vulva to be of normal size, but mainly hidden by folds of adjacent skin
❏ careful inspection of the vulva is often impossible in the conscious animal because of the discomfort it causes
❏ an exudative dermatitis may develop in the skin folds surrounding the vulva; this is exacerbated by the bitch licking the area and by urine scalding
❏ conservative treatment consists of parenteral corticosteroids and antibiotics or locally applied anti-inflammatory creams; application of the latter is usually not well tolerated
❏ permanent treatments involve surgical ablation of the diseased skin and vulval lips with eradication of the sulci around the vulva (see 27.6)

Transmissible venereal tumour (Fig. 14.2)

❏ occasionally seen in the UK around ports
❏ the tumour is caused by seeding of neoplastic cells which are transmitted during coitus
❏ verucose tumours arise in and around the genital tract
❏ they may be removed surgically or the bitch can be treated with a cytotoxic agent, e.g. vincristine

14.2 VESTIBULE

Congenital constrictions

❏ these can occur just inside the vulval lips; they can be dilated digitally or surgically under general anaesthesia

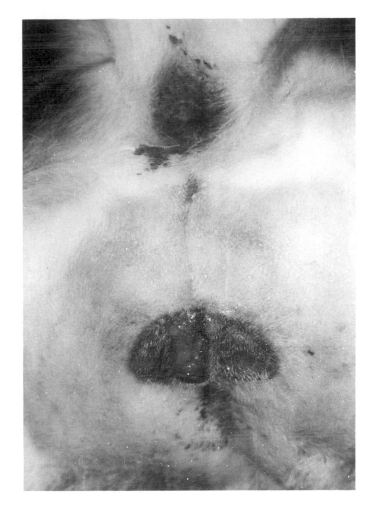

Fig. 14.1 Perivulval dermatitis. Severe inflammation of the vulva and perivulval skin fold.

Enlargement of the clitoris

❏ this may occur either congenitally (see intersexuality) or due to administration of androgens (see 16.4 and 24.3)
❏ frequently the clitoris develops an os, and this causes pain when the bitch sits down, or causes a vestibulitis resulting in excessive licking

Lymphoid hyperplasia (small nodules)

❏ these are sometimes seen in the mucosa; it is suggested that they are caused by a virus, but they do not affect fertility (see 14.3 and 15.1)

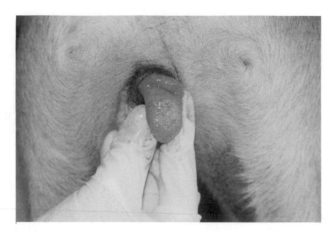

Fig. 14.2 Transmissible venereal tumour affecting the vestibulo-vulva.

14.3 VAGINA

Strictures/stenosis

❏ usually occurs at the vestibulo-vaginal junction, just cranial to the urethral opening
❏ may cause vulval pruritus, vestibulitis and incontinence
❏ simple constrictions appear to be remnants of the hymen and can easily be stretched under general anaesthesia
❏ some constrictions are more resistant to stretching and may continue forward into the vagina as a vertical median fold; these may be difficult to correct surgically, even via an episiotomy (see 27.4)
❏ five aetiologies have been described:
  (a) the result of hypoplasia of the genital canal which causes vestibulo-vaginal hypoplasia and a vaginal stricture of some length
  (b) the result of poor or inadequate fusion of the Müllerian ducts to the urogenital sinus causing annular fibrous strictures at this site
  (c) tissue vestiges remaining at the vestibulo-vaginal junction resulting in hymenal remnants or a complete hymen
  (d) incomplete fusion of the two Müllerian ducts which may result in a double vagina or a vertical fibrous division within the vagina
  (e) imperfect joining of the genital folds and genital swellings resulting in vestibulo-vulval hypoplasia
❏ the extent and position of these lesions may be determined by contrast radiographic examination of the vagina

Vaginal hyperplasia (protrusion) (Fig. 14.3)

❏ occurs in late pro-oestrus and early oestrus when the vaginal wall has become hyperplastic

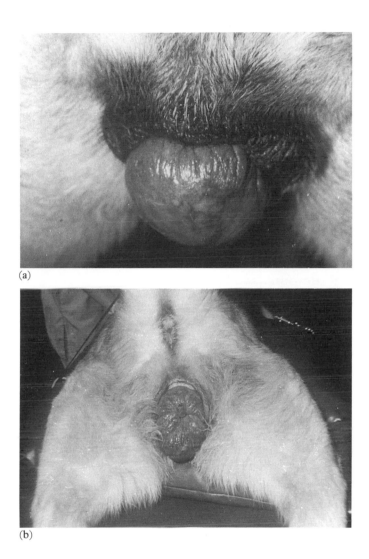

(a)

(b)

Fig. 14.3 Vaginal hyperplasia and protrusion: (a) protrusion of the floor of the vagina; (b) protrusion of the whole circumference of the vagina.

- ❏ it is not clear why this occurs in some bitches and not others
- ❏ in some bitches it first occurs at the first oestrus, in others at a later oestrus
- ❏ once it has occurred, it tends to recur at successive heats
- ❏ the whole circumference of the vagina may protrude; more commonly, however, it is just the vaginal floor
- ❏ the condition may cause urinary incontinence due to prolapse of the urethral opening caudally

Treatment

❏ conservative treatment to reduce trauma is followed by spontaneous resolution after the end of oestrus
❏ ovarohysterectomy (see 25.3) will prevent recurrence of oestrus and therefore prolapse
❏ bitches intended for breeding find mating difficult – the dog tends to introduce his penis ventral to the tissue (Fig. 14.3) and not into the vaginal cavity
❏ surgical removal must be carried out during oestrus, when the full extent of the protrusion can be seen; visualization and control of haemorrhage is easiest if an episiotomy is performed first; care must be taken not to damage the urethra (see 27.5)
❏ the bitch can be mated at the oestrus following surgery; recurrence of the condition is uncommon but can occur

Vaginal tumours (see 27.3)

❏ these only occur in entire bitches
❏ they are usually benign (fibromata, fibroleiomata, etc.) and are often called polyps because they are pedunculated
❏ presenting signs are appearance of the polyp at the vulval lips, or haemorrhage due to ulceration of the surface
❏ surgical removal is usually feasible but may require episiotomy (see 27.2)
❏ occasionally malignant tumours occur under the vaginal epithelium; they most commonly originate in the urethra

Vaginitis (see 4.5, and Fig. 4.1r and s, p. 21)

Definitions

❏ distinguishing between normal and abnormal vulval discharge can be difficult
❏ identifying the source of vulval discharge can be difficult
❏ defining vaginitis in the bitch is almost impossible because all bitches have a normal bacterial flora and have neutrophils in the vaginal smear (except during oestrus)

Causes of vaginal discharge

Normal: pro-oestrus, oestrus, metoestrus, pregnancy, parturition and postpartum

Abnormal: juvenile vaginitis, transmissible venereal tumour, ulcerated polyps, urethral tumours, vaginal trauma, vaginal foreign body, cystitis, pyometra, fetal death, placental separation, post-partum metritis and sub-involution of placental sites

Urinary: ectopic ureter, post-spay incontinence, cystitis, urethral tumours

Diagnosis

❏ in many cases the cause is obvious
❏ vaginal smears will distinguish pro-oestrus and oestrus from other causes (4.5)
❏ bacteriological swabs are of limited value (4.5)
❏ vaginoscopic examination is difficult (4.7)
❏ contrast studies may reveal constrictions, tumours, foreign bodies and ectopic ureters

Prepubertal or juvenile vaginitis

❏ may occur as early as 8 weeks of age
❏ often a copious creamy discharge
❏ no generalized signs of malaise
❏ may contain the normal bacterial flora or very few bacteria
❏ often more epithelial cells than neutrophils in the smear
❏ cause unknown
❏ does not respond to antibiotics, or may improve transiently
❏ may respond to small doses of oestrogen; these may be administered topically or less preferably orally
❏ resolves at pro-oestrus and does not recur

Canine herpes virus

❏ this is probably not a cause of clinical disease in adult bitches
❏ experimental infection causes eruptive lesions on the external genitalia which usually resolve within 7 days
❏ lymphoid hyperpasia (see 14.2 and 15.2) may be a chronic form of canine herpes virus infection but this is not certain

14.4 CERVIX

❏ lesions of the cervix are rare
❏ tumours occasionally occur but are usually asymptomatic

14.5 UTERUS

Aplasia

❏ this is uncommon
❏ if normal uterus is proximal to an aplastic portion, accumulated secretions can cause considerable enlargement of the uterus, which is usually asymptomatic
❏ aplasia of one entire horn is called uterus unicornis
❏ aplasia will cause sterility if it affects the uterine body, or both horns
❏ most cases are found at routine ovariohysterectomy

Cystic endometrial hyperplasia (Fig. 14.4)

❏ during metoestrus (dioestrus) progesterone causes a thickening of the endometrium and massive development of the endometrial glands (see 1.6)
❏ during anoestrus both these changes subside and there is some desquamation of epithelial tissue; however, the endometrium remains thicker than it was before puberty
❏ with succeeding cycles there is progressive permanent thickening of the endometrium and uterine glands become distended (cystic)
❏ cystic endometrial hyperplasia causes no clinical signs; grossly the uterus is thickened (1 cm or more in diameter) and appears to be twisted (Fig. 14.4a)

(a)

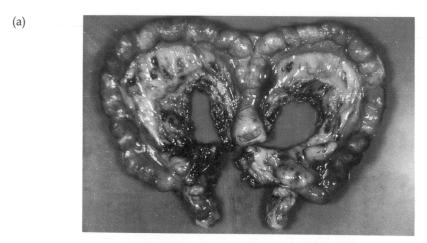

(b)

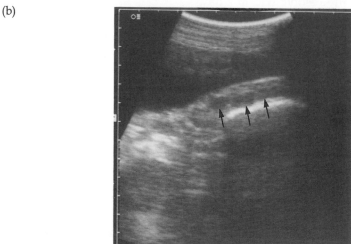

Fig. 14.4 (a) Cystic endometrial hyperplasia; the uterus appears grossly twisted, but there is no exudate in the lumen and no inflammatory reaction. (b) Ultrasound image of the uterine body adjacent to the bladder containing distinct fluid filled cystic regions (arrows) 5.0 MHz transducer; scale in centimetres.

❑ cystic endometrial hyperplasia may, however, be associated with infertility
❑ the condition can be diagnosed using real-time ultrasound examination during the luteal phase (Fig. 14.4b)
❑ treatment is unrewarding, although progesterone receptor antagonists may be useful in the future

Endometritis

❑ there is no convincing evidence that 'low grade' endometritis causes clinical signs in the bitch

Pyometra (Fig. 14.5)

Aetiology

1. During estrus bacteria enter uterus
2. Prog. ↓ immune response
3. Bact. growth → WBC → exudate → pyometra → toxin absorption → toxemia → PU /PD

❑ the vagina has a normal resident bacterial flora (see 4.10)

E. coli

❑ during oestrus the cervix relaxes and these bacteria are able to enter the uterus, especially during mating
❑ usually the defence mechanism of the uterus is competent at eliminating these bacteria, or some mechanism in the cervix (possibly mucus) may prevent their entry
❑ however, if bacteria do enter the uterus, the elevated blood progesterone concentrations at this time may reduce the speed of the inflammatory response (as in other species)
❑ in particular however, bitches with cystic endometrial hyperplasia, i.e. older bitches, seem unable to eliminate these bacteria which may survive in the cyst fluid
❑ the growth of bacteria in the uterus eventually stimulates accumulation of inflammatory exudate, including polymorphonuclear leucocytes
❑ the organism usually isolated from these cases is *Escherichia coli* some strains of which may be more pathogenic than others; streptococci, etc. may also be present
❑ some cases of pyometra are said to be sterile; this may be related to the time of investigation, or because the samples collected were incorrectly handled before culture
❑ accumulation of pus in the uterus is eventually followed by the absorption of bacterial toxins into the circulation and signs of toxaemia
❑ there is no relationship between irregular oestrous cycles and the development of pyometra
❑ there is no relationship between pyometra and pseudo-pregnancy, although both may occur at the same time (see 2.7)
❑ whether or not bitches which have never had a litter are more likely to develop pyometra is not known
❑ the administration of synthetic progestogens may, as does endogenous progesterone, predispose to pyometra by causing cystic endometrial hyperplasia and by directly decreasing the resistance of the endometrium to bacterial invasion (see 24.1)

(a)

(b)

(c)

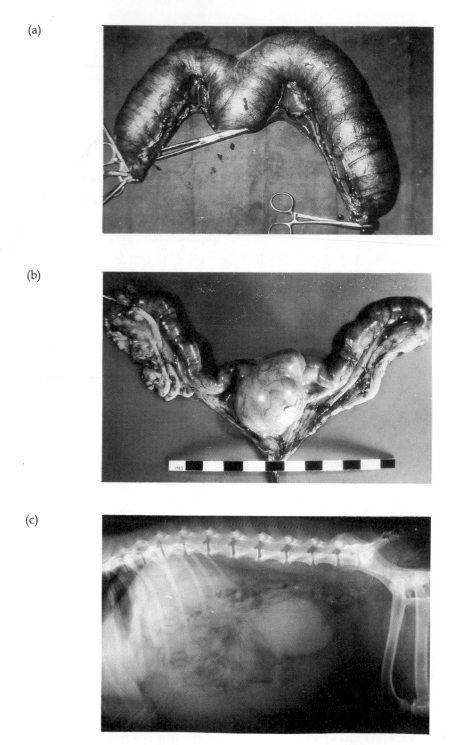

Fig. 14.5

(d)

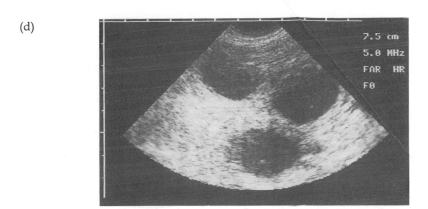

Fig. 14.5   (a) Pyometra causing uniform enlargement of the whole uterus. (b) Pyometra causing partial dilation of the uterus. (c) Lateral radiograph of a bitch with pyometra; note that the enlarged uterus has displaced the colon dorsally and the small intestine cranially. (d) Ultrasound image of a uterus distended with pus. Three sections of the uterine horn are visible containing fluid with small echogenic particles; 5.0 MHz transducer; scale in centimetres.

❑ administration of oestrogens to prevent conception (see 24.2) may predispose to pyometra by keeping the cervix relaxed for longer into the luteal phase than would normally be the case, and allowing bacterial colonization of the uterus

Clinical signs

❑ initially there may be slight pyrexia and depression, but since signs of malaise are vague they are often not noticed
❑ sometimes the appearance of a purulent discharge at the vulva may precede signs of toxaemia, but usually the reverse is true
❑ toxaemia causes varying degrees of depression, anorexia, vomiting, polydipsia, polyuria and occasionally posterior paresis; when presented the body temperature may be normal or subnormal
❑ suppression of erythropoiesis may also occur due to toxaemia
❑ some cases of pyometra are closed, i.e. presumably the cervix is closed and does not allow the escape of pus; in most, however, there is release of exudate although most is retained in the uterus
❑ the relationship between whether pyometra is 'open' or 'closed' and the location of pus in the uterus is unclear; in some bitches only one horn or part of one horn may be distended, in others the whole uterus is equally involved, and in a few there are discrete circular distensions separated by constrictions of the uterus, as in mid pregnancy
❑ in some bitches the distended uterus causes obvious abdominal enlargement

Diagnosis

☐ <u>purulent vaginal discharge</u> accompanied by clinical signs of malaise 4–6 weeks after oestrus is suggestive; however, the signs of toxaemia may develop before or after this

☐ haematology will reveal a <u>neutrophilia</u> (usually in excess of 20×10^7/litre) with a 'shift to the left'

☐ radiography may identify a distended uterus causing dorsal displacement of the colon and cranial displacement of the small intestine; this must be distinguished from pregnancy (see 12.6)

☐ real time ultrasonography will usually reveal a fluid-filled tubular viscus, devoid of fetal elements; the cranial uterine horn may also be imaged above the caudal part

☐ palpation of the abdomen may detect uterine enlargement

☐ mammary development does not preclude the possibility of pyometra because this condition and pseudo-pregnancy are likely to occur at the same time (see 2.7)

☐ laboratory tests may exclude other causes of polydipsia/polyuria, vomiting and paresis

[handwritten: U/S: uterus filled w/ fluid]

Surgical treatment

☐ <u>ovariohysterectomy</u> (see 25.5) is the treatment of choice if the bitch has a reasonable chance of survival; fluid therapy to rehydrate and antibiotics to prevent peritonitis are not optional

Medical treatment

<u>Prostaglandins</u>

[handwritten: 25 mEq/kg BID for 7 days — no side effects c̄ this dosage (0.025 mg/kg) — may be used in closed pyometra, risk uterine rupture / abortion]

☐ medical treatment with prostaglandin $F_{2\alpha}$ has been successful in causing cervical relaxation, myometrial contraction, lysis of corpora lutea and a reduction in plasma progesterone concentration

☐ naturally occurring prostaglandins must be used at low doses (0.25 mg/kg daily or 0.125 mg/kg twice daily for 5 days) to reduce their side effects which include salivation, vomiting, diarrhoea, dyspnoea, abdominal pain and tachycardia *[handwritten: dose too high]*

☐ synthetic prostaglandins are more potent and should be used with care

☐ longer treatment periods are necessary in some cases

☐ prostaglandins are not recommended for use in cases of closed-cervix pyometra because of the risk of uterine rupture

☐ broad spectrum antimicrobial therapy should always be administered because 10% of bitches with pyometra are bacteraemic *[handwritten: *broad spectrum antibiotics for 3 wks]*

☐ a return to fertility may occur in approximately 20% of bitches

☐ long term complications include recurrent metritis, anoestrus, failure to conceive and abortion

[left margin handwritten notes: open pyometra — often mistaken as a vaginitis; closed pyometra: toxemia (dep pyrexia, PU/PD) no reacts, uterus filled w/ fluid]

Progesterone receptor antagonists

❑ RU46534 has been investigated in bitches with pyometra
❑ administration on days 1, 3, 5, 8 and 16 after presentation was successful for the treatment of pyometra in the majority of dogs
❑ the regime produced no adverse effects, and emptying of uterine fluid occurred quickly, producing resolution of the clinical signs
❑ some of the bitches returned to normal fertility after treatment

NB: if medical treatment is successful, it is likely that the condition will recur following the next oestrus; it may therefore be prudent to plan to breed the bitch at the first oestrus after treatment

Metorrhagie

❑ post-oestrus bleeding is seen in some old bitches
❑ the bitch is often assumed still to be in oestrus by the owner
❑ examination reveals that the discharge is dark and unlike that in normal oestrus
❑ there are no signs of malaise attributable to the condition
❑ a diagnosis of pyometra is often made, although this is erroneous
❑ ovariohysterectomy is however the only treatment
❑ the removed uterus is slightly enlarged and the ovaries contain 'cystic' structures; these may be adenomata although the aetiology of the condition requires further investigation

Uterine tumours

❑ uterine tumours are uncommon
❑ leiomyomata are seen in older bitches
❑ they are rarely associated with clinical signs

14.6 UTERINE TUBES

❑ lesions are rare; occasional tumours occur

14.7 OVARIES

Ovarian cysts

❑ cystic follicles and corpora lutea are uncommon and are not usually associated with clinical signs
❑ occasionally follicular cysts result in persistent oestrus; these can be diagnosed by ultrasonographic imaging
❑ occasionally luteal cysts result in a delayed return to oestrus; these may be diagnosed by a persistently raised plasma progesterone concentration
❑ neither cyst can be treated by the exogenous use of hormones

❑ cysts of the tubular elements of the ovary and adjacent tissues are less rare and are encountered during routine ovariohysterectomy; they cause no clinical signs

Ovarian tumours

❑ granulosa cell tumours are usually associated with persistent or recurrent oestrus; both plasma oestrogens and progesterone concentrations are reported to be elevated
❑ adenomata (cyst adenomata) may affect both ovaries and are normally benign; their possible association with metorrhagie (see 14.5) is unclear
❑ diagnosis may be made on the basis of clinical signs, palpation, radiography, ultrasonography and plasma steroid assay
❑ the presence of ovarian tumours, particularly dysgerminomata and teratomata, may also be suspected if abdominal distention occurs
❑ surgical removal is usually effective unless metastases have occurred
❑ care should be taken not to rupture these neoplasms since metastatic spread is often by trans-coelomic seeding

15 Abnormalities of the Reproductive Tract of the Dog

15.1 PREPUCE (SHEATH)

Phimosis

- ❏ this is constriction of the preputial orifice such that the penis cannot be exteriorized
- ❏ it may occur congenitally or as the result of trauma or inflammation
- ❏ in severe cases urine cannot escape as it is voided; it accumulates in the sheath and dribbles thereafter from the preputial opening
- ❏ affected dogs are not able to copulate and show signs of pain during erection
- ❏ surgical enlargement of the orifice is usually curative (27.11)

Paraphimosis

- ❏ this occurs when the penis can be exposed from the sheath, but cannot be retracted
- ❏ it is not always an absolute disparity between the size of the preputial orifice and the size of the penis
- ❏ in some dogs after normal copulation the penis is slow to return to the sheath, or causes inversion of the preputial skin and hair; lubrication of the penis with a water soluble gel will aid its return, although the dog may resent manipulation of the penis – failure to help causes paraphimosis
- ❏ spinal lesions can cause paraphimosis
- ❏ foreign bodies may cause paraphimosis
- ❏ if the erect penis cannot be detumified, it soon becomes dry and cyanotic; the application of ice packs and lubricants under general anaesthesia may be required to reduce swelling
- ❏ subsequent surgical enlargement of the preputial orifice may prevent recurrence (see 27.11)
- ❏ on occasions the exact cause of the condition is unclear and correction may involve amputation of the engorged penis (27.13)

Priapism

- ❏ this is persistent enlargement of the penis in the absence of sexual excitement
- ❏ it may be the result of neurogenic abnormalities such as lumbar spinal lesions
- ❏ conservative management may be successful, although some cases require penile amputation

Short pepuce

❏   these, and those with abnormally positioned orifices, are usually associated with intersexuality (see 16.4)

Balanitis

❏   this is inflammation of the lining of the sheath (see balanoposthitis)

Persistent protrusion of the penis

❏   in some otherwise normal male dogs the tip of the penis protrudes from the sheath
❏   it is not clear whether the prepuce is too short or the penis too long
❏   protrusion may be permanent, or may only occur when the dog sits
❏   often the condition causes no problem, but sometimes drying of the mucosa and self trauma necessitate treatment
❏   operations to pull the prepuce forward are usually unsuccessful
❏   amputation of the distal penis may be necessary (see 27.13)

Urination on the chest and front legs

❏   seen in some King Charles spaniels
❏   despite 'cocking' a hind leg, urine is usually deposited on the ventral thorax and back of one or both front legs
❏   this causes problems for the owner who either has to wash the dog several times a day or 'put up with' the smell
❏   the cause is unknown
❏   operations to pull the prepuce forward and thus deviate the urine ventrally are rarely effective
❏   amputation of the distal penis (27.13) allows the now empty prepuce to direct the urine away from the body

15.2 PENIS

Penile hypoplasia

❏   extremely rare but reported in certain breeds
❏   may be due to sex chromosome abnormalities
❏   the clinical signs are related to urine pooling within the prepuce

Hypospadias

❏   this is opening of the urethra somewhere along the ventral surface of the penis, and not at its tip; it may be as far back as the anus
❏   six classifications have been described, of which the perineal form is the most common
❏   invariably this condition occurs in intersexual dogs (see 16.4)

❑ affected dogs may also have a short and deviated penis
❑ reconstructive surgery or amputation may be required

Persistent frenulum

❑ this is a band of tissue attaching the ventral surface of the penis to the adjacent prepuce
❑ this frenulum has usually disappeared by puberty
❑ if it persists, attempts to extrude the penis from the repuce may cause pain, ventral deviation of the penis or haemorrhage if the frenulum ruptures
❑ surgical section of the frenulum under general anaesthesia may be necessary (see 27.12)
❑ a heritable nature has been established in one breed

Haemorrhage

❑ haemorrhage through the penile integument may occur apparently spontaneously or after known trauma, e.g. dog bite
❑ torn areas of integument rarely heal well
❑ mattress sutures of fine absorbable material should be used to occlude the lesion under general anaesthesia
❑ if lesions are refractory to this treatment, the penis should be amputated and the dog castrated (in order to try to avoid the dog obtaining an erection)

Fracture of the os penis

❑ usually causes urethral haemorrhage and perhaps dysuria
❑ diagnosis is by palpation and radiographic examination
❑ treatment initially is to allow healing to occur unaided
❑ indwelling urethral catheters may be useful during the initial healing phase
❑ if callus formation causes urethral constriction, penile amputation or perineal or scrotal urethrostomy should be considered

Lymphoid hyperplasia

❑ this is diagnosed when many 1–2 mm raised nodules are noticed towards the base of the glans penis
❑ the condition has wrongly been called 'dog pox'; the lesions are not vesicles
❑ the cause may be viral but there is no evidence of clinical disease or coital spread (14.3)
❑ lesions are often found incidentally during routine fertility examination; their significance is not known
❑ occasionally these nodules may be abraded during mating or semen collection

Posthitis

❑ this is inflammation of the penis; it is rare but areas of congestion-like discolouration are sometimes seen – the cause is unknown

❑ dogs with excessive purulent discharge from the prepuce are often said to have balanoposthitis (inflammation of the penis and sheath) but
(a) all entire male dogs have some discharge from the prepuce
(b) close inspection of the penis and sheath usually reveals no sign of inflammation
(c) swabs and smears of the surface of the penis will reveal macrophages, polymorphonuclear leucocytes and bacteria, which are all normal
(d) ureoplasmata and mycoplasmata are normal in the dog prepuce and semen

Preputial discharge

❑ some preputial discharge is normal; it may drip from the prepuce or be licked away by the dog (Fig. 15.1)
❑ it is difficult to define *excessive* discharge; this may depend on the dog's owner, i.e. what is acceptable in a kenneled dog may not be acceptable in a dog which sits on furniture
❑ there is no known cause in dogs which do not have obvious lesions, e.g. foreign bodies
❑ during routine fertility examinations, quite copious accumulation of pus may be seen with or without lymphoid hyperplasia and are considered normal
❑ bacteriological culture frequently reveals normal commensal organisms
❑ culture of an antibiotic resistant bacterium, e.g. *Pseudomonas aeruginosa* or any other organism in pure culture, may be significant, but this occurs very rarely
❑ parenteral treatment with antibiotics is usually not necessary and is not effective

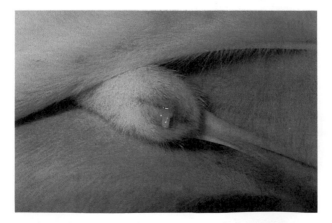

Fig. 15.1 Photograph of the sheath of a dog showing a normal volume of preputial discharge which may drip from the prepuce or be licked away by the dog.

❏ parenteral treatment with sex steroids to reduce sexual activity and self interest may help; if so, castration may be a permanent cure

❏ flushing the prepuce (general anaesthesia may be necessary) with intra-mammary antibiotic preparations or weak antiseptic solutions may be effective but repeat treatments are usually necessary. This treatment may select for other organisms and should be avoided if at all possible

NB: pus may originate from the prostate gland but the dog invariably shows other signs of prostate disease (see 15.7). Reduction in pus production by the normal prepuce/penis may be impossible because it is probably stimulated by as yet unidentified factors

Penile neoplasms

❏ tumours of the penis are rare

❏ squamous cell carcinomas are the most usual type and commonly spread locally and metastasize to inguinal lymph nodes

❏ haemorrhage from an ulcerated neoplasm may be the first clinical sign

❏ in the absence of metastases radical surgical resection is warranted

Transmissible venereal tumour

❏ coitally transmitted neoplasm that spreads by 'seeding' of infected cells

❏ lesions are usually friable, ulcerated and often haemorrhagic (Fig. 15.2)

❏ the tumour is not normally found within the UK

❏ local excision, amputation and chemotherapy may be suitable treatments depending upon the location and extent of the tumour

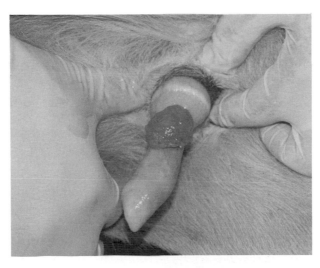

Fig. 15.2 Photograph of the penis of a dog showing the presence of a tumour-like mass that was subsequently found to be a transmissible venereal tumour. Such lesions are usually friable, ulcerated and often haemorrhagic.

15.3 TESTES

Anorchia (anorchism)

❑ congenital absence of both testes
❑ there is only one documented case of a male dog being born without testicles
❑ can be confirmed by a lack of response to a human chorionic gonadotrophin (hCG) stimulation test (see 4.11)

Monorchidism

❑ this is the condition of a dog having only one testicle
❑ it has not been reported as a congenital condition but can exist after surgical removal of one testis
❑ it should not be confused with unilateral cryptorchidism

Cryptorchidism

❑ this is a condition in which there is failure of one or both testes to pass through the inguinal ring (see 5.7) and enter the scrotum
❑ depending on whether both or one testicle fails to descend, the dog is called a bilateral or unilateral cryptorchid (*not* monorchid)
❑ testes which are in the abdomen produce testosterone (see 7.4) but not spermatozoa (see 6.1)
❑ unilateral cryptorchids are usually fertile but bilateral cryptorchids are not
❑ cryptorchids usually have normal libido
❑ testes are normally descended by 10 days of age but may be difficult to palpate in young pups due to their small size and the presence of scrotal fat; therefore a diagnosis is usually not confirmed until 10 weeks of age
❑ bilateral cryptorchids can be diagnosed by a positive responce to an hCG stimulation test (see 4.11)
❑ as cryptorchid dogs get older, the chance of normal descent becomes more remote; it is very rare after 1 year of age
❑ sometimes fully descended testes in pups appear to become abdominal again; the reason for this is not known
❑ there is no reliable medical treatment
❑ in any event, medical treatment is not ethical since the condition has a genetic base
❑ the mode of inheritance is not fully known but it follows the model of a sex-limited autosomal recessive trait:
  (a) both female and male parents will carry the gene
  (b) homozygous males will be cryptorchid
❑ treatment is removal of the abdominal testis surgically (see 27.10) because these testes are more likely to become neoplastic than scrotal testes
❑ removal of the other testis at the same time is desirable to prevent the dog from breeding

❏ surgical removal of the abdominal testis is not necessary until 18 months of age, as neoplastic changes are unlikely before this time

Ectopic testes

❏ these are testes which do not occupy a normal scrotal position
❏ the abdominal testes of cryptorchid dogs are therefore ectopic
❏ testes which have passed through the inguinal canal may then migrate away from the scrotum to become ectopic
❏ these testes may be found:
(a) anterior to the scrotum, under the skin and lateral to the penis; these may be palpated under the skin
(b) in the femoral triangle; these are not palpable
(c) caudally in the perineum, lateral to the corpus cavernosum; these may be palpable
❏ treatment is as for cryptorchid dogs (see 27.10)

Hypoplasia

❏ scrotal testes which do not develop properly, i.e. remain small after birth, are rare; small testes are usually the result of degeneration

Traumatic orchitis (inflammation of the testis)

❏ this may occur during any incident, but is commonly the result of dog fights
❏ conservative therapy includes local cleansing, antibiosis, diuretics to reduce swelling and measures to prevent self trauma
❏ deep testicular lesions rarely heal well and may necessitate castration
❏ healing is often followed by degeneration

Non-traumatic orchitis

❏ inflammation of the testis is rarely proven to occur due to haematological spread, or ascending infection from the urinary tract
❏ *Brucella canis* infection does not occur in the UK; it causes acute orchitis and epididymitis with sperm abnormalities – treatment is difficult (see 19.5)
❏ orchitis can be associated with autoimmune thyroiditis
❏ some dogs which show no clinical signs of disease of the testes or prostrate glands produce ejaculates containing large numbers of inflammatory cells (see 9.5); their origin is unknown (the surface of the penis must be eliminated as the source)

Testicular torsion

❏ this is more correctly torsion of the spermatic cord
❏ the cause of the torsion is unknown
❏ as a result of the torsion the pampiniform plexus (see 5.6) becomes compressed but blood continues to enter the testis via the spermatic artery; this

causes rapid swelling and usually pain such that the dog is reluctant to move; on occasions palpation of the testis is not resented
❏ there is swelling of the pampiniform plexus, epididymis and testis (Fig. 15.3)
❏ frequently there is self trauma to the scrotum because of the pain
❏ haematuria may be a presenting sign
❏ diagnosis is easy in scrotal testes
❏ torsion of an abdominal testis produces acute abdominal pain, the cause of which may only be diagnosed at exploratory laparotomy
❏ surgical removal of the affected testis gives rapid pain relief and is always warranted as the testis will never function properly again

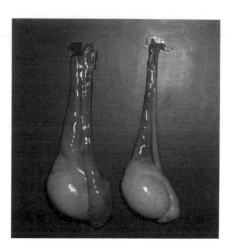

Fig. 15.3 Photograph of the scrotal contents of a dog following castration. In one there was torsion of the spermatic cord, resulting in swelling of the pampiniform plexus, epididymis and testis. The contralateral testis is normal.

Testicular degeneration (atrophy)

❏ affected testes are small, hard and the surface may be uneven
❏ usually both the spermatogenic and endocrine functions of the testis are lost:
  (a) plasma testosterone concentrations are low
  (b) plasma LH and FSH concentrations are high
❏ it is the known sequel of orchitis and testicular torsion

Abnormal spermatogenesis (see 9.5)

❏ this is the cause of some abnormal ejaculates (see 9.5) associated with infertility
❏ the affected testes may be normal, soft or small
❏ the condition may be permanent for unknown reasons, or temporary, as caused by pyrexia (see 5.6) and some drugs (see Chapter 24)
❏ there may be increased or decreased echogenicity of the testicular parenchyma when examined with ultrasound

❏ diagnosis may, however, require fine needle aspiration or testicular biopsy
NB: there is no evidence that vaccination against parvovirus disease causes infertility in dogs

Spermatogenic arrest (see 9.5)

❏ this is a specific testicular degeneration
❏ affected dogs are usually fertile initially
❏ spermatogenesis stops suddenly, often between 18 months and 7 years of age
❏ semen collection shows the presence of prostatic fluid and no spermatozoa
❏ the dog shows no signs of malaise
❏ the testes may be smaller and softer than normal
❏ the condition is irreversible
❏ it is probably an autoimmune disease
❏ it is inherited in some breeds
❏ diagnosis can be made on the basis of semen evaluation, changes in testicular ultrasonographic appearance, fine needle aspiration, and testicular biopsy
❏ early on in the disease process many abnormal spermatozoa may be found within the ejaculate

Relationship of semen quality to fertility

Normal semen quality

❏ on average semen quality is superior in fertile compared with non-fertile samples
❏ however, there is no unimpeachable method of predicting the fertility of a semen sample
❏ 'normal values' from a variety of breeds are given in Table 15.1
❏ some dogs with poor semen quality may be fertile using assisted reproductive techniques

Table 15.1 Characteristics of the second fraction of the ejaculate from 53 fertile dogs.

	Motility (%)	Volume (ml)	Concentration ($\times 10^6$/ml)	Total sperm output ($\times 10^6$)
Mean	85.2	1.3	310.5	403.4
S.D.	6.2	0.4	82	120
Range	42–92	0.4–3.4	50–560	36–620
	Live normal (%)	Dead normal (%)	Primary abnormal (%)	Secondary abnormal (%)
Mean	75.2	10.2	1.6	10.0
S.D.	7.9	5.4	2.6	5.4
Range	52–90	2–26	0–12	2–24

Spermatozoal number

❑ an inverse relationship has been established between ejaculate volume and spermatozoal concentration

❑ there are also differences between large and small breeds of dog

❑ the determination of the total number of spermatozoa per ejaculate is the most accurate measure of sperm production

❑ infertility in the dog has not been associated simply with reduced spermatozoal numbers, although irreversible azoospermia in previously fertile dogs has been recognized for some time

❑ cases of functional azoospermia with spermatogenic arrest have been recorded in two related Welsh springer spaniels and in some related labrador retrievers

❑ one case of azoospermia has been reported which was reversed following sexual rest

❑ a seasonal effect on spermatozoal production has been noted in dogs in warm climates

Spermatozoal morphology

❑ a high incidence of morphologically abnormal spermatozoa is often associated with reduced fertility

❑ there have been few reports concerning the influence of specific morphological abnormalities on fertility

❑ abnormal mid piece droplets were identified in an infertile greyhound dog

❑ abnormal head–base/mid piece regions have also been associated with infertility
(a) the commonest abnormality was swelling of the mid piece region
(b) electron-microscopic studies showed axonemal and mitochondrial defects both within these membrane swellings and at other regions of the mid piece

❑ spermatozoa with mid piece defects and deformed acrosomes have been found associated with experimental *Brucella canis* infection

❑ no other spermatozoal morphological abnormalities have been reported to affect fertility in the dog

❑ however, the relationship between the percentage of morphologically abnormal spermatozoa and fertility of the dog has recently been established:
(a) the fertility of dogs with greater than 60% morphologically normal spermatozoa was 61%
(b) the fertility for those with less than 60% morphologically normal spermatozoa was 13%

Vital staining

❑ staining of spermatozoa with a vital stain is considered part of the normal morphological assessment

- ❑ in several species there have been good correlations found between the percentage of vital staining spermatozoa and fertility
- ❑ there are two factors that may be involved:
    (a) the effect of the total number of live spermatozoa on fertility
    (b) the interference with fertility by the proportion of dead spermatozoa
- ❑ in the dog there has been little study of the proportion of dead spermatozoa within the ejaculate; commonly only the total number of morphologically normal live staining spermatozoa are considered

Spermatozoal motility

- ❑ some workers have suggested that spermatozoal motility is the best predictor of male infertility
- ❑ human sperm swimming speeds correlate well with the results of *in vitro* fertilization assays
- ❑ to date there are no similar studies in dogs, but there is no doubt a relationship between motility and fertility

Cytological studies

- ❑ in man much importance has been given to the presence of cells other than spermatozoa within the ejaculate
- ❑ little attention has been given to the presence of these cell types in the dog
- ❑ it is common for inflammatory cells to be noted within the ejaculate; however, these frequently originate from the prepuce

Assessment of spermatozoal function

- ❑ traditional criteria of semen quality are based upon descriptive assessments of ejaculate characteristics
- ❑ however, fertile dogs have been reported with low numbers of normal spermatozoa
- ❑ the phenomenon of spermatozoal swelling in the presence of hypo-osmotic medium has been investigated

Treatment of dogs with poor semen quality

- ❑ most medical treatments are unrewarding and the owner should be given realistic advice before embarking on therapy
- ❑ the anti-oestrogens, clomiphene citrate and tamoxifen, may be useful in some cases:
    (a) these agents are antagonists at the hypothalamic receptor level; they displace oestrogen from the receptor and lead to a decreased negative feedback of the oestrogen
    (b) as a result gonadotrophin release is increased
    (c) the enhanced secretion of LH and FSH may stimulate spermatogenesis and Leydig cell function
    NB: clomiphene has significant intrinsic oestrogenic activity which may

directly impair spermatogenesis; tamoxifen has no such oestrogenic activity and may be more suitable
❏ an analogue of dihydrotestosterone, mesterolone, is unusual in that it is not aromatized to oestradiol and therefore, at therapeutic doses, does not significantly suppress the release of pituitary gonadotrophins; it may be useful for stimulating spermatogenesis and it has been used in dogs, but its effects have not as yet been fully evaluated

General points on infertile dogs

❏ 'overuse' is rarely a cause of infertility; most dogs produce sufficient spermatozoa for two fertile ejaculations per day
❏ if semen quality is poor, allow the dog to mate twice daily for as long as the bitch will stand
❏ if there has been recent illness (pyrexia) it is prudent to rest the dog for 2 months. This is not because this will allow recuperation, but because the ejaculate will probably be abnormal for this length of time
❏ do not use androgens (testosterone or its esters) in dogs with poor semen quality or poor libido; these are very likely to suppress spermatogenesis
❏ parvovirus vaccination does not cause infertility in male dogs
❏ the probable success of thyroid hormone supplementation is low

Hydrocoele/spermatocoele

❏ these are very rare in the dog
❏ they may be diagnosed by palpation and ultrasound imaging
❏ they are the result of outflow obstruction

Testicular tumours

❏ testicular tumours are the second most common tumour affecting the male dog

Sertoli cell tumours

❏ these are discrete, slow growing and often unilateral
❏ they cause testicular enlargement
❏ they usually produce oestrogen which causes feminization (attractive to male dogs, gynaecomastia, pendulous prepuce, bilateral non-pruritic alopecia, see 24.2)
❏ may cause bone marrow suppression
❏ rarely metastasize; only 10% are malignant
❏ spermatogenesis stops in both testes; the unaffected testis atrophies due to the indirect effect of oestrogen on the pituitary gland
❏ high oestrogen concentrations may cause bone marrow suppression and squamous metaplasia of the prostate gland
❏ small endocrinologically active tumours may cause clinical signs but be non-palpable; these tumours may be diagnosed ultrasonographically

❏ should be removed surgically by castration (see 26.3 and 27.14); unilateral castration may result in a return to fertility once the negative feedback effect of oestrogen has been removed

Seminomas (seminomata)

❏ arise from spermatogenic tissue of the tubular epithelium
❏ are usually solitary and unilateral
❏ cause testicular enlargement
❏ usually hormonally inactive
❏ sometimes metastasize
❏ spermatogenesis stops and feminization may occur
❏ should be removed surgically

Interstitial cell tumours

❏ arise from Leydig cells
❏ may be single or multiple in one or both testes
❏ 1–2 cm in diameter
❏ yellow in colour when sliced open
❏ affected testicles may shrink due to loss of seminiferous tubules
❏ spermatogenesis stops
❏ usually hormonally inactive (surprisingly)
❏ often not diagnosed due to lack of clinical signs and lack of clinical importance
NB: diagnosis of Sertoli cell tumours and seminomata in abdominal testes may only be at exploratory laparotomy by which time metastasis may have occurred

Feminizing syndrome (see also 17.4)

❏ this is sometimes seen in dogs with grossly normal testes; castration cures the condition (see 26.3)
❏ this also occurs in some castrated dogs, and adrenal steroid production has been implicated
(a) may be diagnosed by detecting elevated concentrations of 17-hydroxy-progesterone following a standard ACTH stimulation test
(b) signs may be controlled by the negative feedback effects of exogenous androgens or progestogens

15.4 EPIDIDYMIDES

❏ trauma and inflammation may occur as in the testis
❏ one case of aplasia has been recorded
❏ idiopathic blockage may occur as in other species, but has not been recorded in the dog
❏ measurement of the epididymal markers alkaline phosphatase and carnitine may be useful for the diagnosis of obstructive azoospermia, but care must be taken to ensure that complete ejaculation has occurred

15.5 VASA DEFERENTIA

❏ idiopathic blockage may occur but has not been recorded
❏ one case of deferential aplasia has been recorded

15.6 URETHRA

❏ hypospadias is usually, but not always, associated with intersexuality (see 15.2 and 16.4)
❏ urethritis is rare *per se* but may be associated with urinary calculi, fracture of the os penis and repeated catheterization (see 15.2)

Urethral prolapse

❏ excessive sexual excitement or urinary straining may produce prolapse of the terminal portion of the urethra
❏ the everted portion becomes oedematous and may bleed
❏ the common presentation is excessive licking at the prepuce
❏ some dogs show no clinical signs
❏ the urethra may be replaced if not damaged
❏ castration should be considered to prevent recurrence
❏ amputation of the distal penis may be necessary when there is marked trauma or the problem is recurrent

15.7 PROSTATE GLAND

Prostatic disease is common in the older entire male dog. Accurate detection and diagnosis of prostatic disease requires the use of many diagnostic tools (see Chapter 9).

Benign prostatic hyperplasia

❏ hyperplasia of the prostatic epithelium begins early in the dog's life
❏ this is associated with altered androgen:oestrogen ratios and may be present without clinical signs
❏ however, in some dogs the enlarged gland impinges on the pelvic viscera and causes:
(a) faecal tenesmus
(b) haematuria
(c) haemospermia
❏ usually the gland is symmetrically enlarged and non-painful
❏ the large gland may be demonstrated radiographically:
(a) a pneumocystogram may be useful for the accurate identification of the gland
(b) positive contrast urethrograms may be useful for the assessment of the position of the urethra, and changes within the prostatic urethra
❏ ultrasonographically there is often enlargement of the gland and slight increased echogenicity:

(a) this change may mask the normal appearance of the hilar echo

(b) the condition may progress to cystic hyperplasia when the gland margin may become irregular

❏ castration produces rapid resolution of clinical signs

❏ exogenous progestogens and oestrogens may also be used to reduce circulating androgen concentrations and therefore reduce prostatic size; these however have little effect on established lesions

NB: oestrogens may induce prostatic squamous metaplasia resulting in increased size of the gland

❏ anti-androgens such as cyproterone acetate, flutamide, finasteride and formestane may be useful for the control of this condition, but whilst all of these anti-androgens are commercially available, non are licensed for use in the dog

Bacterial prostatitis

❏ adult dogs may develop prostatitis following ascending infection of bacteria, commonly *Escherichia coli*

❏ the condition is sometimes a sequel to hyperplasia

❏ clinical signs include systemic illness, with vomiting and caudal abdominal pain

❏ dogs are frequently neutrophilic and the gland is painful and has an irregular contour on palpation

❏ culture of the third fraction of the ejaculate, urethral washing or urine may help with diagnosis

❏ patchy focal echogenic regions may be identified with ultrasound but early ultrasonographic findings may be equivocal

❏ lesions may become chronic, and pockets of purulent exudate may form (prostatic abscessation) producing signs of recurrent cystitis

❏ treatment of these cases is difficult; antimicrobial therapy on the basis of the results of bacterial sensitivity may be required for up to 6 weeks

❏ in certain cases surgical drainage is necessary

Squamous prostatic metaplasia

❏ a change in the prostatic glandular epithelium from cuboidal or columnar to squamous occurs secondarily to endogenous or exogenous hyperoestrogenism (e.g. Sertoli cell tumours)

❏ this change predisposes to cyst formation, infection and abscessation, but is not a pre-neoplastic change

❏ a presumptive diagnosis may be made on the history and clinical signs

❏ treatment is directed towards removal of the source of oestrogen because the condition is reversible

Prostatic cysts

❏ two types of prostatic cyst have been identified

❏ the least common are discrete retention cysts associated with blockage of the

prostatic ducts; these occur within the parenchyma of the prostate, causing distortion of its outline
❑ more commonly, cysts are found adjacent to the prostate (paraprostatic cysts), attached by small stalk-like adhesions; these are remnants of the uterus masculinus
❑ the clinical signs of both types of cyst are related to their size; they may produce pelvic canal obstruction, faecal tenesmus, dysuria and haematuria
❑ diagnosis may be made radiographically, although ultrasound examination can differentiate the internal architecture of the organ:
(a) paraprostatic cysts are frequently large anechoic structures positioned cranial or dorso-cranial to the bladder
(b) the removal of urine or injection of small volumes of air into the bladder may allow differentiation from the paraprostatic cyst in cases of doubt
(c) the cyst wall can be of variable thickness and may be echogenic due to calcification
(d) cyst fluid may contain echogenic material which often sediments to the dependent portion
(e) many cysts have echogenic internal septae and a connection to the prostate gland may sometimes be imaged
(f) it is not uncommon for cystic lesions to also be identified within the prostate gland (Fig. 15.4)
❑ excision or marsupialization are the treatments of choice; castration and hormone therapy are of no value

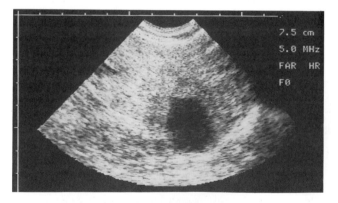

Fig. 15.4 Ultrasound image of a dog with a 2 cm diameter intra-prostatic cyst of no clinical significance; 5.0 MHz transducer, scale in centimetres.

Prostatic neoplasia

❑ adenocarcinomata are the most common neoplasms affecting the prostate gland of the dog (Fig. 15.5)
❑ tumours are firm upon palpation and tend to metastasize to iliac and sublumbar lymph nodes and to the vertebral bodies of caudal lumbar vertebrae

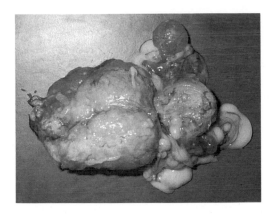

Fig. 15.5 Prostatic adenocarcinoma.

❑ clinical signs are associated with the increased size of the gland, although dogs may have a haemorrhagic urethral discharge and hind-limb pain
❑ diagnosis may be made on the basis of clinical signs, radiographic findings, the presence of neoplastic cells collected by urethral washing following prostatic massage or semen collection
❑ patchy focal regions of mixed echogenicity may be identified with ultrasound; these may be associated with an increased parenchymal echogenicity and fine echogenic speckles
❑ fine needle aspiration under ultrasound guidance or biopsy are valuable diagnostic tools
❑ the animal should be carefully examined for metastatic spread before embarking on therapy
❑ treatment can be palliative by the administration of oestrogens, anti-androgens, and by castration

Medical therapy for prostatic disease (see also Chapter 24)

❑ long term therapy is aimed at reducing the size of the gland, i.e. reducing circulating concentrations of androgens
❑ this can be achieved by the repeated administration of hormone preparations:
   (a) oestrogens which have a negative feedback effect upon the pituitary but suffer the risk of inducing prostatic metaplasia
   (b) progestogens which have a negative feedback effect upon the pituitary (cyproterone acetate is often used in man)
   (c) flutamide which inhibits androgen uptake and/or nuclear binding of androgen
   (d) finasteride a specific 5 α reductase inhibitor which prevents the conversion of testosterone to dihydrotestosterone
   (e) formestane which is an aromatase inhibitor which inhibits the conversion of androgen to oestrogen in peripheral tissue
❑ or, by castration

NB: neither therapy will produce permanent relief of large prostatic cysts or neoplasia

❏ antibiotics which are chosen for chronic prostatitis and prostatic abscessation should be chosen upon the basis of specific sensitivity; however, ery-thromycin, chloramphenicol and trimethoprim are most likely to be con-centrated in prostatic fluid, although other agents may penetrate the gland when it is inflamed
❏ analgesics and anti-inflammatory drugs may be indicated
❏ surgical removal of the whole gland, a portion of the gland, a cystic region of abscessated area may be considered

Effects of prostatic disease on fertility

❏ blood and inflammatory cells in the ejaculate do not seem to affect fertility
❏ treatment with oestrogens and progestagens will inhibit testicular and pro-static function temporarily; after treatment fertility may return but so may clinical signs of disease
❏ castration and prostatic removal cause sterility

15.8 SCROTUM

Scrotal trauma (abrasions, eczema)

❏ this is painful and generally exacerbated by the dog licking
❏ immediate treatment (antibiotics, analgesics, Elizabethan collar) should prevent testicular changes associated with a local increase in temperature (see 6.2)

Inguinal (scrotal) hernia

❏ this is rare in the dog and is recognized as swelling in the scrotum due to the passage of abdominal contents through the inguinal canal
❏ treatment is surgical correction, castration and closure of the inguinal canal

16 Intersexuality

Intersexuality is usually recognized because of abnormal phenotypic sex appearance.

16.1 DEFINITIONS

True hermaphrodite: in mammals this word is used to describe individuals which have both testicular and ovarian tissue; invariably the testicular tissue is intra-abdominal so that spermatogenesis does not occur

Male pseudohermaphrodite: this is an animal with testicular tissue but external genitalia which are to a greater or lesser extent 'female-like' (Fig. 16.1a)

Female pseudohermaphrodite: has ovarian tissue but external genitalia which are to a greater or lesser extent 'male-like' (Fig. 16.1b)

Intersex: this is an individual in which the physical features do not conform to those generally recognized as belonging to the male or female: this is the best word to use to describe dogs of indeterminate sex as their gonadal content will not be known until histological examination is made

16.2 AETIOLOGY

Intersex animals may be classified into those with abnormalities of chromasomal, gonadal or phenotypic sex

Abnormalities of chromosomal sex

Recognition of chromosomal abnormalities requires construction of a karyotype

- ❑ generally these animals are phenotypic males or females with under-developed genitalia
- ❑ not usually an inherited condition
- ❑ can be an extra sex chromosome, e.g. XXY, XXX
- ❑ can be only one sex chromosome, e.g. XO
- ❑ can be a mosaic, i.e. more than one cell line in the same individual with different sex chromosome contents, e.g. XX/XY or XX/XXY

Abnormalities of gonadal sex

- ❑ where chromosomal and gonadal sex do not agree, the animal is said to be 'sex-reversed'

❏ only XX sex reversal is seen in dogs, i.e. XX male or XX pseudo-hermaphrodite
❏ such dogs have testes or ovotestes
❏ an inherited condition of cocker spaniels and other breeds
❏ thought to be caused by an inherited sex-reversal gene

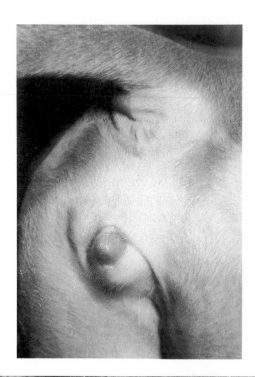

(a)

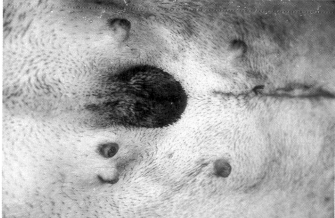

(b)

Fig. 16.1

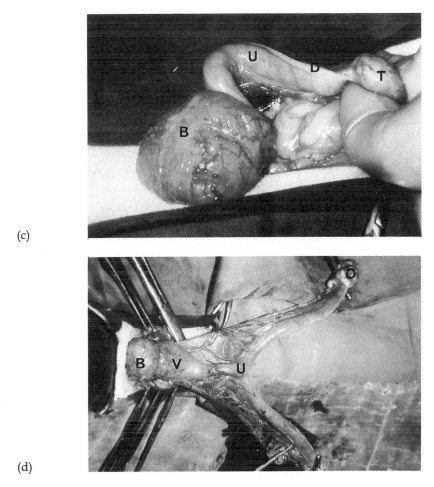

(c)

(d)

Fig. 16.1 Intersexual dogs: (a) this animal was sold as a normal female pup; at 5–6 months of age, growth and exposure of the phallus (clitoris) was noticed; (b) this dog was assumed to be a normal male until he was presented with haemorrhage from the prepuce and a history of being attractive to male dogs; closer examination revealed that the prepuce was rudimentary, there was no palpable penis and the dog was in oestrus; (c) internal genitalia from dog in (a); a uterine horn (U), ductus deferens (D) and testis (T) are shown (B, urinary bladder); (d) internal genitalia from dog in (b); the vagina (V), uterus (U) and ovaries (O) are shown (B, urinary bladder).

Abnormalities of phenotypic sex

❏ gonadal and chromosomal sex agree, but external genitalia are intermediate
❏ female pseudohermaphrodites are caused by exposure to sex steroids (usually androgens or progestogens) *in utero*
❏ male pseudohermaphroditism may be inherited or be due to a defect in androgen production

16.3   CLINICAL SIGNS

❑   affected individuals are usually not recognized as puppies
❑   commonly, abnormal development of the genitalia, particularly enlargement of the clitoris (phallus), is noticed at about 6 months of age
❑   other signs which alert an owner to abnormality are pro-oestrous bleeding in dogs thought to be males, and urinary incontinence
❑   incontinence is usually caused when a normal vagina opens into a severely narrowed vestibule associated with an enlarged os clitoridis (Fig. 16.1); urine is then voided normally from the bladder but accumulates in the distended vagina from which it leaks slowly via the stenosed vestibule
❑   adult dogs, particularly male pseudohermaphrodites, may first be presented with pyometra or Sertoli cell tumour

16.4   EXTERNAL PHYSICAL SIGNS

❑   in dogs that look mainly female, the vulva is more ventrally placed than usual and may be between the thighs; there may be varying protrusion of the clitoris due to enlargement of the *os clitoridis* which now resembles a small *os penis* with a narrowed vestibular canal running like a male urethra along its caudal surface
❑   in dogs that look mainly male-like the preputial opening is further forward but the prepuce is short; the preputial opening may be ventral with urethral hypospadias (see 15.2) – alternatively the prepuce may be normal but contains no penis
❑   if testicles are present in either of the above they may be abdominal or scrotal

16.5   INTERNAL REPRODUCTIVE ORGANS

❑   irrespective of the external signs the gonads may be ovaries, testes or a mixture of both (ovotestes); they may be in a normal ovarian position, or located anywhere along the normal testis path of descent
❑   irrespective of the sort of gonads present, the tubular genitalia may consist of a uterus, or epididymis/vas deferens, or both together

16.6   TREATMENT

❑   intersexual dogs are nearly always sterile
❑   removal of the gonads and tubular genitalia at laparotomy (see 27.10) prevents the discomfort that some animals show in oestrus and avoids pyometra and testicular tumours
❑   after removal of testicular tissue from dogs with a protruding phallus, time should be allowed for this to regress; otherwise reduction of the size of the phallus by removing the os clitoridis/penis may be necessary
❑   there may be no cure for incontinence in intersexual dogs

17 Abnormal Bitch Physiology and Endocrinology

17.1 DELAYED PUBERTY (PRIMARY ANOESTRUS)

- ❏ the age of a bitch at her first pro-oestrus/oestrus is very variable; it may not occur until she is over 2 years of age
- ❏ the reason for this delay is usually not known
- ❏ when pro-oestrus/oestrus does eventually occur, it is usually normal
- ❏ there is no reason why a mature bitch should not be mated at her first oestrus
- ❏ plasma progesterone concentration should be measured. An elevated concentration indicates that the oestrus has been missed by the owner
- ❏ if oestrus has not been missed and the delay is causing concern, oestrus-induction may be attempted (see 17.5)
- ❏ if signs of pro-oestrus/oestrus are induced this at least confirms that the bitch has an ovary and that it can respond to gonadotrophic stimuli
- ❏ a dog with X-chromosome trisomy and elevated follicle stimulating hormone (FSH) and luteinizing hormone (LH) plasma concentrations has been reported; it was still anoestrus at 4 years old
- ❏ hypothyroidism is rarely thought to cause primary anoestrus

17.2 PROLONGED FIRST PRO-OESTRUS

- ❏ in some bitches the first pro-oestrus does not proceed to oestrus and may last for 3 weeks or more, or pro oestrus may terminate and recur some weeks later
- ❏ presumably there is insufficient pituitary stimulation to cause follicle maturation
- ❏ ovulation does not occur, follicles therefore regress and signs of pro-oestrus disappear
- ❏ theoretically, administration of human chorionic gonadotrophin (hCG) should caused ovulation; this is rarely effective which suggests that follicles are still immature
- ❏ often a second follicular phase appears (2–12 weeks later) and the bitch ovulates normally
- ❏ when the signs of pro-oestrus are very prolonged and hCG treatment has been unsuccessful megestrol acetate (2 mg/kg) for 8 days usually causes cesation of pro-oestrus; the time of occurrence of the next pro-oestrus is variable but it usually then proceeds normally

17.3 PROLONGED PRO-OESTRUS OR OESTRUS

❑   a condition similar to 17.2 may occur in the adult bitch that has previously been normal
❑   management is as described above

17.4 SHORT INTER-OESTROUS PERIODS (OVULATION FAILURE)

❑   intervals of less than 4 months between successive oestrous periods suggest that:
    (a) ovulation (luteinization) may not have occurred (see 2.4)
    (b) the luteal phase may be short; this has only been reported after oestrus induction
❑   anovulation occurs in approximately 1% of oestrous cycles
❑   confirmation of ovulation can be achieved by monitoring plasma progesterone concentrations
❑   the length of the luteal phase can be monitored by regular measurement of plasma progesterone concentration (see 21.4)
❑   in cases of anovulation, an attempt to induce ovulation can be made by the administration of hCG, but
    (a) it is difficult to know when to administer this
    (b) early administration may result in follicular luteinization
    (c) late administration may be ineffectual

17.5 PROLONGED ANOESTRUS

❑   the inter-oestrous interval may normally be longer than expected:
    (a) the cause of this is unknown but may relate to seasonal influences
    (b) if these delays interfere with a breeding programme, oestrus induction may be considered (see 21.4)
❑   a common problem is the failure to observe the signs of oestrus; elevated concentrations of progesterone (greater than 2 ng/ml) will indicate missed ovarian activity within the previous 2 months
❑   prolonged anoestrus represents an inter-oestrus interval greater than anticipated for that particular animal
❑   there is limited evidence of a role of hypothyroidism in the delayed return to oestrus, but investigating thyroid function is rarely rewarding
❑   progesterone-producing ovarian cysts have been described in the bitch, producing prolonged inter-oestrous intervals and cystic endometrial hyperplasia; these may be identified using ultrasonography or radiology and the diagnosis confirmed by serial measurement of plasma progesterone concentration
❑   drug-induced anoestrus should also be considered; preparations that have the ability to prevent oestrus include progestogens, androgens, glucocorticoids and anabolic steroids
❑   oestrus induction may be attempted if there is no underlying disease and if breeding is essential

17.6 UNPREDICTABLE OVULATION TIME (see also 2.4

- ❏ whilst the 'average bitch' ovulates approximately 12 (of pro-oestrus, this is not true for all bitches:
    - (a) some bitches ovulate as early as day 5 after the onset of p₁.
    - (b) some bitches ovulate as late as day 30 after the onset of pro-oestru.
- ❏ such bitches are normal but they are not 'average'
- ❏ bitches are not necessarily consistent at successive heats; some bitches may vary by as much as 12 days in the day of ovulation between successive cycles, i.e. they ovulate on day 8 at one oestrus and day 20 at the subsequent oestrus
- ❏ careful monitoring of each oestrous cycle is therefore warranted; this can be achieved using vaginal cytology, vaginal endoscopy, and measurement of plasma progesterone concentration

17.7 SILENT OESTRUS

- ❏ some bitches have normal cyclical activity, including follicular growth and ovulation, without any external signs of pro-oestrus or oestrus
- ❏ certain breeds, for example the greyhound, may have only slight sero-sanguinous discharge and minimal vulval swelling during oestrus
- ❏ ovulation may be confirmed by examination of plasma progesterone concentration
- ❏ alternatively, the weekly collection of cells from the bitch's vagina will allow anticipation of oestrus

17.8 PSEUDOPREGNANCY (see also 2.7)

- ❏ many non-pregnant bitches exhibit signs which are similar to those seen normally during the pre-partum and post-partum periods
- ❏ signs may develop occasionally, or following every oestrus in an individual bitch
- ❏ the clinical signs of pseudopregnancy are not associated with any endocrine abnormality; they are related to a normal elevated plasma concentration of prolactin
- ❏ the term physiological pseudopregnancy may be used in some cases, because in every non-pregnant bitch there is some degree of mammary gland enlargement

Clinical signs

- ❏ clinical pseudopregnancy (sometimes referred to as overt pseudopregnancy) has a variable clinical presentation including anorexia, nervousness, aggression, nest making, nursing of inanimate objects, lactation and occasionally false parturition
- ❏ in some cases lactation may result in mastitis

❑ pseudopregnancy is generally noted between 6 and 12 weeks after the end of oestrus, during the decline in plasma progesterone concentration

❑ it may also occur should plasma progesterone concentration decline for other reasons:

(a) removal of the ovaries (i.e. ovariohysterectomy) during the luteal phase will result in a rapid reduction in plasma concentration of progesterone, and a subsequent rise in plasma concentration of prolactin

(b) lysis of the corpora lutea may result in a rise in plasma prolactin concentration, i.e. following spontaneous abortion in late pregnancy, or the pharmacological termination of pregnancy

❑ in many cases pseudopregnancy undergoes spontaneous remission, especially if there is no stimulus for continued lactation (no sucking)

❑ in some cases either the physical or the psychological signs, or the effect of these signs upon the owner, may warrant treatment of the condition

❑ in some cases pseudopregnancy may persist for many months, or even several years; the reason for this is unknown, but presumably relates to a lack of hormonal interaction between the pituitary/hypothalamus and the ovary

❑ is often mistakenly stated that clinical pseudopregnancy predisposes to pyometra, infertility and ovarian abnormalities; however, this is not the case

Treatment

❑ in the majority of cases, clinical pseudopregnancy requires no treatment; spontaneous resolution can be allowed to occur

❑ ovariohysterectomy has no value for the treatment of clinical pseudo-pregnancy:

(a) at certain stages of the cycle removal of the ovaries will cause a further reduction in plasma progesterone, and potentiate the rise of plasma pro-lactin

(b) ovariohysterectomy will prevent the occurrence of pseudopregnancy, but caution should be exercised in performing surgery too soon after recovery

(c) in bitches that have repeated clinical pseudopregnancy the best time to perform surgery is during the subsequent oestrus

Conservative treatment

❑ sedative agents may be useful, but phenothiazines may be inappropriate, because they are dopamine antagonists and may produce a rise in prolactin concentration

❑ massage of the mammary glands should be avoided because stimulation may potentiate a further rise in prolactin concentration

❑ diuretic agents may speed the resolution of the clinical signs but should be administered with care, especially if the bitch is anorexic

Drug therapy

Progestogens

❏ progesterone (or progestogens) rapidly reduces the clinical signs
❏ this probably works by suppression of pituitary release of prolactin
❏ progestogens may be administered either orally daily (e.g. megestrol acetate), or by depot injection (e.g. proligestone or delmadinone acetate)
❏ first generation progestogens such as medroxyprogesterone acetate are not recommended because they might potentiate the development of a pyometra
❏ oral therapy is often associated with relapse of the clinical signs, if therapy is terminated too quickly

Oestrogens and androgens

❏ oestrogens and androgens, and combinations of these steroids, are effective at reducing the clinical signs of clinical pseudopregnancy
❏ their mechanism is likely to be the same as that of progesterone
❏ androgens or oestrogens are not frequently used alone; however, a synthetic androgen, mibolerone, which is not available in the UK but is available in the USA, is effective
❏ combinations of ethinyl oestradiol and methyltestosterone are commercially available to treat clinical pseudopregnancy in the bitch:
  (a) the response is usually good
  (b) the risk of adverse effects is low
NB: oestrogens may produce bone marrow suppression, and androgens may produce clitoral enlargement and aggression, although when used in combination the individual drug doses are reduced and the risk of adverse effects is low

Prolactin antagonists

❏ several synthetic ergot alkaloids (dopamine agonists) have been shown to be inhibitors of prolactin secretion
❏ bromocriptine has been used for some time to reduce prolactin concentrations and control the signs of clinical pseudopregnancy:
  (a) it is not specific in its action and oral administration causes vomiting in a large number of bitches
  (b) these effects can be reduced by starting with a very low dose and increasing this gradually over several days
  (c) vomiting may be reduced by mixing the drug with food, or by the prior administration of metoclopramide, although the latter does not make pharmacological sense because bromocriptine and metoclopramide have opposing dopaminergic actions
❏ cabergoline also reduces the plasma concentration of prolactin, and whilst it is not presently available in the UK it is widely available in Europe; it has a higher activity, longer duration of action, better tolerance, and produces less vomiting than bromocriptine

17.9 THYROID DEFICIENCY

❑ hypothyroidism is said to cause infertility occasionally in the bitch
❑ this may be via a delayed return to oestrus
❑ lymphocytic thyroiditis has been identified as a cause of infertility in beagles and borzois
❑ thyroid supplementation may improve fertility although this is disputed by many workers

17.10 OTHER HORMONAL ABNORMALITIES

❑ to date there have been few descriptions of hormone abnormalities which cause unusual behaviour or conditions in the bitch because:
(a) the only hormones readily measured in the bitch are progesterone and oestrogen
(b) hormonal changes are so rapid that frequent sampling would be necessary but impracticable; the assay of single samples is usually worthless (except progesterone, see 21.4)
❑ terms such as 'ovarian imbalance' and 'hormonal imbalance' are meaningless because they cannot be defined

Conditions sometimes said to be caused by hormonal abnormalities

Mounting and thrusting behaviour

❑ this occurs in both entire and neutered bitches
❑ it may be more marked when other oestrous bitches are present
❑ there is no evidence that it is caused by an excess of androgens or any other specific hormone change
❑ it can be controlled by training

Urine marking

❑ during pro-oestrus and oestrus it is common for bitches to pass small volumes of urine frequently; they may also urinate on vertical objects
❑ bitches may also do this when not in oestrus and even after neutering; it does not indicate a hormonal anomaly

Urinary incontinence (see 25.6)

❑ this may occur in older bitches which have been neutered
❑ such bitches do not have lower oestrogen concentrations than other neutered bitches (within the limits of sensitivity of the assays available)
❑ the reason why only some neutered bitches are affected is not known
❑ many bitches respond to low dose oestrogen therapy (see 24.2)

Oestrogen responsive dermatosis

❑ some neutered bitches develop a bilateral, non-pruritic alopecia, usually with hyperpigmentation of the skin
❑ if response to thyroid replacement therapy is poor, oestrogen treatment may be effective (see 24.2)
❑ such bitches cannot be said to be hypo-oestrogenic because plasma concentrations are in the same range as other neutered bitches

Unwillingness to mate during oestrus

❑ some bitches which are considered to be in oestrus by virtue of vaginal and other changes (see 4.5) will not allow mating
❑ hormone concentrations have not been reported but are probably within the normal range
❑ the condition is usually psychological and seen in bitches which have had little contact with other dogs
❑ treatments include tranquillizers, exposure to a different male dog and artificial insemination

18 Abnormal Dog Physiology and Endocrinology

18.1 HYPOGONADISM

- ❏ reduced secretion of follicle stimulating hormone (FSH) and luteinizing hormone (LH) may occur in cases of pituitary dysfunction and will result in impaired spermatogenesis
- ❏ serial blood sampling demonstrates that plasma LH, FSH and testosterone concentrations are low
- ❏ testicular biopsy demonstrates an absence of spermatogenesis but no inflammation
- ❏ the administration of FSH has been suggested to promote spermatogenesis although the efficacy of this technique remains to be proven

18.2 POOR LIBIDO

- ❏ frequently, inability to copulate is the result of inexperience on behalf of the dog or poor breeding management
- ❏ there is no evidence that reduced libido is the result of low plasma androgen concentrations
- ❏ the administration of exogenous androgens is rarely curative, and can have an inhibitory effect upon pituitary function
- ❏ in man, exogenous androgens have been shown to reduce gonadotrophin secretion, resulting in the suppression of endogenous testosterone secretion and testicular activity

18.3 IMPAIRED SPERMATOGENESIS

- ❏ differing terminology has been used to describe an absence of spermatogenesis, including primary testicular failure, primary failure of spermatogenesis and Leydig cell failure
- ❏ little is known about the occurrence and true aetiology of these conditions and inappropriate terminology has been frequently adapted from other species
- ❏ low plasma concentrations of FSH and LH may indicate a hypothalamic or pituitary lesion
- ❏ normal or increased concentrations of FSH and LH are suggestive of primary spermatogenic failure with loss of feedback inhibition
- ❏ low concentrations of plasma LH, FSH and testosterone may also occur secondarily to thyroid hormone deficiency

❑ histologically, the testes of many azoospermic dogs have tubular degeneration, with normal or sparse numbers of Leydig cells
❑ certain cases of oligospermia may respond to the administration of oestrogen analogues (clomiphene citrate) or anti-oestrogen compounds (tamoxifen); it has been suggested that these cases represent early stages of primary spermatogenic failure
❑ the synthetic androgen, mesterolone, may also be useful
❑ thyroid function should always be evaluated in cases of poor semen quality: cases of hypothyroidism may benefit from supplementation; however, the prognosis for fertility is often poor

18.4 OTHER CAUSES OF ABNORMAL SPERMATOGENESIS

❑ testicular trauma resulting in both tissue damage and elevated temperature
❑ testicular tumours resulting in reduced normal spermatogenesis and endocrine changes
❑ testicular ectopia resulting in increased testicular temperature
❑ systemic hyperthermia
❑ aplasia of testis or epididymis
❑ scrotal trauma or eczema resulting in elevated temperature
❑ testicular degeneration after orchitis, torsion, or other inflammatory conditions
❑ autoimmunity resulting in spermatogenic arrest
❑ unknown causes of spermatogenic arrest
❑ edogenous endocrine disturbances:
   (a) testicular tumours
   (b) pituitary tumours rarely affect fertility
   (c) raised FSH and LH plasma concentrations have been reported in dogs with spermatogenic arrest
❑ exogenous hormone therapy: progestogens, oestrogens and androgens inhibit pituitary release of gonadotrophins and interfere with spermatogenesis; such therapy may have been given to reduce sex drive and fertility or to control prostatic disease

18.5 IMPAIRED SPERMATOZOAL TRANSPORT

Accelerated passage through the epididymis

❑ this may account for the occasional finding of large numbers of immature spermatozoa in the ejaculate – these have proximal cytoplasmic droplets (see 9.5); the cause is unknown

Retrograde ejaculation

❑ this is the forward movement of spermatozoa along the urethra and into the bladder, which occurs in man and may occur in dogs; it is common to find

spermatozoa in dog urine and this is probably due to the expulsion of unejaculated sperms
❑ sperm present within the bladder are often immotile, but may return to motility and fertility after washing
❑ the condition may be due to an incompetent bladder sphincter and treatment may be attempted using sympathomimetic agents
❑ in man a 10% success has been reported using the tricyclic antidepressant agents which have significant anticholinergic effects

Prostatic disease

❑ the effect of prostatic disease on sperm transport and the composition of prostatic fluid is unknown, as is their influence on seminal quality

Synthetic glucocorticosteroid therapy

❑ this has a rapid deleterious effect on semen quality which is probably mediated in the epididymis

18.6 IMPOTENCE (INABILITY TO COPULATE) (see also 18.2 and 21.5)

Causes

❑ inexperience
❑ fear: chastisement for mounting behaviour in young dogs may be remembered when dogs are subsequently used at stud
❑ pain: particularly prostatic, penile or skeletal pain; in these cases the dog will appear to be interested in a bitch in oestrus but will not be able to mount, gain intromission or achieve a 'tie'
❑ endocrine anomaly: there is no evidence that reduced testosterone production is a cause of impotence, or that testosterone therapy is curative
NB: it is often impossible to make a specific diagnosis in cases of impotence

18.7 ATTRACTIVENESS TO OTHER MALE DOGS

❑ this occurs occasionally, usually years after castration
❑ no hormonal cause has been identified, but circulating testosterone concentrations would be expected to be low
❑ can also be caused by oestrogen-producing testicular tumours (see 15.3)
❑ pheromones appear to be produced but do not seem to originate in the anal sacs or prepuce
❑ testosterone therapy may be effective in some cases, and depot preparations or prolonged oral administration is required

19 Pregnancy Failure

19.1 FERTILIZATION FAILURE

- ❏ the most common cause is an inappropriate mating time (see 8.2 and 10.1)
- ❏ may be the result of poor semen quality
- ❏ may follow the use of cryopreserved semen which has a short longevity in the female tract
- ❏ rarely, anovulation may occur (see 17.4)
- ❏ administration of oestrogens will prevent conception
- ❏ unknown factors including abnormal oocytes or abnormalities of the female reproductive tract may prevent conception

19.2 EARLY EMBRYONIC DEATH

- ❏ the rate and time at which this occurs is not known
- ❏ individual embryos may fail to develop due to genetic abnormalities
- ❏ whole pregnancies may fail due to cystic endometrial hyperplasia or the persistence of bacteria in the uterus, although this has not been conclusively proven

19.3 RESORPTION

- ❏ it has long been suspected that some established and diagnosed pregnancies fail without signs of abortion
- ❏ recently, the use of real time ultrasound has confirmed this (Fig. 19.1)
- ❏ resorption may occur when the pregnancy fails before day 35
- ❏ after embryonic/fetal death the fluids are resorbed into the bitch's circulation and the tissues (membranes and embryo/fetus) become dehydrated and autolysed
- ❏ at laparotomy uteri have been seen where there is evidence of resorption of one or two conceptuses (Fig. 11.1, p. 77)
- ❏ spontaneous resorption of one or two embryos appears to occur in up to 10% of pregnancies
- ❏ in these cases the remaining pregnancy continues and normal pups are born at term
- ❏ on occasions the whole litter can be resorbed
- ❏ the cause is frequently not known, but is probably not due to a progesterone deficiency:
  - (a) it may be a mechanism for reducing the number of conceptuses
  - (b) some infectious agents may cause resorption
  - (c) chromosomal abnormalities may account for some conceptual losses

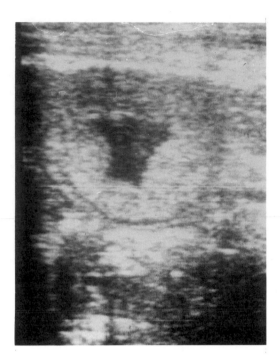

Fig. 19.1   Isolated embryonic resorption in a bitch. There is loss of the normal spherical outline, inward bulging of the conceptual wall and increased echogenicity of the yolk sac fluid. Five normal conceptuses were also present and these were delivered normally at term; 7.5 MHz transducer.

19.4 BODY PREGNANCY

❏   occasionally a conceptus develops in the body of the uterus
❏   after about 25–30 days, blood from the marginal haematoma starts to escape
❏   if bleeding is severe, complete ovariohysterectomy should be considered
❏   alternatively, the body pregnancy may be expelled spontaneously
❏   ideally, the viability of the remaining pregnancies is monitored using real-time ultrasound

19.5 ABORTION

Bacterial causes of abortion

Brucella canis *infection*

❏   not seen in the UK but some dogs with antibodies to the organism have been identified
❏   abortions usually occur after the 30th day
❏   may also cause early resorption
❏   generalized lymph node enlargement is common in the bitch

❑ aborted material (and semen from males) is highly infectious
❑ bacteriaemia may persist for years
❑ response to treatment is poor
❑ affected animals should never be used for breeding

Miscellaneous bacteria

❑ may be present in the uteus after mating, but may also enter via the cervix in later pregnancy
❑ the bitch usually expels all fetuses and membranes
❑ the fetal stomach is the best place to sample for bacteriology; bacteria found here were ingested *in utero*
❑ broad spectrum antibiotic treatment for aborting bitches is prudent until results of bacteriology are known
❑ generalized malaise or infectious disease is rarely associated with abortion
❑ abortions tend to be sporadic, but occasionally several bitches in a kennels are affected
❑ organisms isolated include *Escherichia coli*, campylobacter, pseudomonas, salmonella, haemolytic streptococci and clostridia
❑ *Brucella abortus* has been known to produce abortion via infected cows' milk, but this is now unlikely in the UK

Viral causes of abortion

Canine herpes virus

❑ in adult dogs generally produces a few mild signs limited to the respiratory or genital tract
❑ the uncomplicated disease may be unnoticed by the owner
❑ genital tract lesions are frequently raised nodules that are red in colour
❑ lesions are evident at the onset of pro-oestrus, suggesting venereal transmission is probably important
❑ recrudescent virus shedding from the vesicular lesions may be stimulated by the stress of pregnancy and parturition
❑ infection in the bitch may be associated with infertility, abortion and stillbirths
❑ infection of the pregnant bitch results in placental lesions and the infection of the fetuses:
(a) infection during early pregnancy may result in fetal death and mummification
(b) infection during mid-pregnancy results in abortion
(c) infection during late pregnancy results in premature birth
❑ pups may become infected at birth, during passage through the vagina, and subsequently die with widespread necrotizing lesions
❑ the source of the virus is oral, nasal or vaginal secretions (and possibly preputial excretions)
❑ pathological changes are often characteristic of canine herpes virus infection, and virus can be isolated readily from these tissues

❏ infection in the adult dog often requires no treatment and the condition is self limiting
❏ in pregnant bitches supportive therapy during the abortion is required
❏ in the pups, the disease is rapidly fatal and treatment is often unrewarding
❏ bitches which have previously given birth to infected pups may later deliver a normal litter
❏ resorbing and aborting bitches should be isolated from other pregnant bitches
❏ infected bedding should be removed and the environment disinfected
❏ the potential for viral transmission at coitus is uncertain; however, males with reproductive tract lesions should not be used for mating

Canine distemper virus

❏ in susceptible dogs a peracute form with sudden onset pyrexia and death may occur
❏ most infections result in primary respiratory tract or gastrointestinal tract signs
❏ some dogs may develop central nervous system lesions
❏ some may develop hyperkeratosis of the pads and nose ('hardpad')
❏ experimental exposure of pregnant bitches produces either:
   (a) clinical illness in the bitch with abortion, or
   (b) subclinical infection of the bitch and the birth of clinically affected pups
❏ diagnosis is via post-mortem, histopathology and virus isolation
❏ there is no suitable treatment for the reproductive tract consequences of distemper virus infection
❏ vaccination is now performed using attenuated live virus vaccines

Canine parvovirus

❏ canine parvovirus 1 has not been confirmed as a major cause of disease
❏ canine parvovirus 2 appears to have arisen as a host range mutant of feline parvovirus
❏ the virus may cross the placenta and affect pups which then develop acute generalized infection and myocardial disease soon after birth
❏ a diagnosis may be made upon the clinical signs, supported by a leuco-paenia, and the identification of virus or viral proteins
❏ the reproductive consequences can be treated by supportive nursing of affected pups, especially using fluid therapy and antimicrobial agents
❏ inactivated canine parvovirus vaccines are available, and recently live tissue culture attenuated vaccines have been selected

Canine adenovirus

❏ canine adenovirus 1 is a highly contagious disease known to produce infectious canine hepatitis
❏ the virus may cross the placenta during late pregnancy, resulting in the birth

of pups which rapidly develop signs of systemic infection similar to those observed in older pups and adults
- ❏ some pups may be born dead whilst others are weak and die within a few days of parturition
- ❏ infection may be diagnosed upon the basis of the clinical signs, and virus isolation
- ❏ adjuvanted inactivated vaccines are available and in certain cases their single administration can provide immunity for life

Protozoal causes

Toxoplasma gondii

- ❏ this has been implicated in canine abortion

Abortion of unknown aetiology

- ❏ endocrine insufficiency may be responsible but has not been identified, although hypothyroidism is a possible cause
- ❏ there is no clear data to show that low plasma progesterone concentrations cause resorption or abortion
- ❏ many bitches which abort habitually have uterine disease such as cystic endometrial hyperplasia; this can be evaluated ultrasonographically
- ❏ ingestion of toxic substances is rarely identified as a cause
- ❏ although there are many potentially teratogenic substances, they are rarely a cause of pregnancy failure in bitches

Partial abortion

- ❏ there are several recorded cases of bitches aborting some pups and having others normally at term
- ❏ the presence of live pups can be confirmed by ultrasound examination
- ❏ antibiotic therapy should be given after abortion to try to prevent bacteria from affecting the other fetuses

NB: tetracyclines should not be given to pregnant bitches as they may cause discoloration of the pups' teeth. Ampicillin and amoxycillin are the safest antibiotics to use during pregnancy

Prevention of abortion

- ❏ in bitches with a history of abortion, the following may be tried:
    (a) broad spectrum antibiosis immediately after mating to reduce bacterial colonization of the uterus
    (b) broad spectrum antibiosis (*not* tetracyclines) at the time of expected abortion in the belief that bacteria enter the uterus via the cervix during pregnancy
    (c) progesterone supplementation in the belief that low progesterone concentrations result in abortion. This has never been proven except following

oestrus-induction regimes. Administration of progesterone or progestogens during pregnancy may delay or prevent parturition, and may cause urogenital abnormalities in the pups

19.6 METROCOELE

❑ rarely the uterus can become trapped in the inguinal ring
❑ if the bitch becomes pregnant a swelling (conceptus) may start to develop in this area
❑ early detection may allow the uterus to be returned to the abdomen surgically
❑ more commonly hysterotomy must be performed, perhaps with hysterectomy

19.7 UTERINE RUPTURE

❑ this may apparently occur asymptomatically
❑ pups which are expelled from the uterus die and become dehydrated (mummified)
❑ they are sometimes discovered during routine examination or laparotomy
❑ may also occur close to term (see 20.9)

19.8 LOSS OF FETAL FLUID

❑ in late pregnancy this occasionally occurs spontaneously when the bitch is suffering a hydrops condition (it is unknown whether this is hydrops amnii or hydroallantois)

20 Dystocia and Post-partum Problems

20.1 DEFINITIONS

Eutocia: normal birth

Dystocia: any problem which interferes with normal birth

Obstructive dystocia: problem with birth which causes unproductive straining; due to malpositioning of a pup, relative fetal oversize or a blockage in the reproductive tract

Primary uterine inertia: absence of uterine contractions and therefore first stage parturition; the cervix relaxes but pups do not enter the vagina and there is no sign of parturition – if untreated the pups die

❏ the cause is unknown but may be due to:
(a) a small number of pups (one or two) producing an inadequate stimulus (?glucocorticosteroids) to initiate complete parturition
(b) a very large litter (or excess fetal fluid – 'hydrops') causing over-stretching of the uterus and preventing myometrial contractions
(c) insufficient calcium (subclinical eclampsia) in the myometrium; this may be related to a dietary insufficiency, inadequate parathyroid hormone or a refractory parathyroid gland (see 13.3 and 20.15)
(d) an unknown endocrinological imbalance or insufficiency
(e) may be inherited

Secondary uterine inertia: cessation of uterine contractions after they have started, presumably due to exhaustion of the myometrium or some of the factors involved in primary inertia
(a) secondary inertia early in second stage parturition usually follows an obstructive dystocia (unproductive straining)
(b) secondary inertia later in second stage parturition may occur apparently spontaneously after the normal birth of several pups. The length of time for which uterine inactivity can be considered normal is impossible to define; however, if treatment results in the birth of a dead pup, secondary inertia can be retrospectively diagnosed

20.2 THE 'OVERDUE' BITCH (see 13.4)

Possible causes

❏ early mating (see 11.1) in relation to the time of ovulation (pregnancy can be as long as 72 days)

❑ inaccurate information or calculation of expected whelping day
❑ primary uterine inertia
❑ non-pregnancy
❑ pregnancy loss, e.g. resorption or abortion

Investigation

❑ check mating date
❑ palpate abdomen (but see 12.4)
❑ auscultate abdomen for fetal heart beats (see 12.5)
❑ radiograph bitch; pups will be observed if she is pregnant but their viability may be unknown. Radiographic signs of fetal death include:
(a) overlapping of the skull bones
(b) accumulation of gas in the fetal stomach or subcutaneously
(c) abnormal fetal posture
(d) additionally, fetal bones in the bitch's stomach may indicate that she has whelped/aborted and eaten the pups
❑ ultrasonography will confirm pregnancy and the viability of those pups which are accessible to the ultrasound beam. Ultrasonographic signs of fetal death include:
(a) absence of fetal heart beat (Fig. 20.1)
(b) absence of fetal movements
(c) reduced volume of fetal fluid
(d) accumulation of gas in the fetal stomach or subcutaneously
❑ measurement of plasma progesterone concentration. Progesterone concentrations decrease 24–36 hours before parturition (Fig. 20.2); detection of high concentrations indicates that parturition is not immiment, whilst basal concentrations indicate that parurition should have begun. ELISA techniques may be useful in the practice laboratory
❑ endoscopic examination. It is not possible to palpate the cervix digitally;

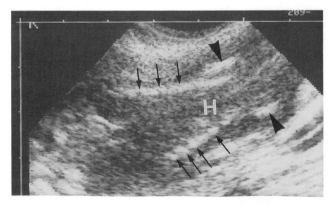

Fig. 20.1 Ultrasound image of a dead fetus *in utero*. The fetal ribs (small arrows) and scapulae (arrow heads) can be seen; however, the fetal heart (H) has stopped moving and no longer appears anechoic; 5.0 MHz transducer, scale in centimetres.

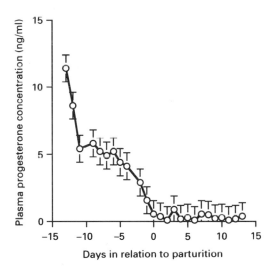

Fig. 20.2 Periparturient changes in plasma progesterone concentration.

however, endoscopic examination may allow inspection of the cervix and cranial vagina

Treatment if pregnant

❏ it may be decided to give the bitch more time if the vagina is dry and tight, especially if the mating history is vague

❏ if dead pups are identified, caesarean operation (oxytocin may be tried first, but is unlikely to work)

❏ if primary inertia is suspected due to temperature fall (see 13.3) more than 48 hours previously, or evidence of placental separation (see 20.3), oxytocin may be tried but caesarean operation is more successful

20.3 HAEMORRHAGIC (BLACK/GREEN) DISCHARGE AT TERM WITH NO SIGNS OF LABOUR

Possible causes

❏ primary uterine inertia with fetal (at least one) death and placental separation: this may be in a bitch known to be pregnant, or often in an aged bitch which was not known to have been mated and has only conceived one pup

❏ death of all the fetuses in mid to late pregnancy followed by haematic mummification; the cause is unknown and the pups may die at different stages of development

Investigation

❏ palpation and auscultation may be useful but are not diagnostic

❑ radiology may confirm fetal death but only several days after it has occurred
❑ ultrasonography is the diagnostic method of choice

Treatment

❑ caesarean operation

20.4 NERVOUS INHIBITION OF LABOUR

❑ in this case the bitch may be in first or second stage labour but will not settle to whelp properly and may have successive pups in different places, or carry them about

Possible causes

❑ bitch being put into unfamiliar place (garage, etc.) to whelp
❑ bitch being introduced to whelping box too close to term
❑ bitch not wanting to be away from her owner and familiar surroundings

Treatment

❑ allow the bitch to whelp where she wants and hope that it is not too inconvenient!
❑ ensure the owner is present until whelping is over
❑ prevent unfamiliar persons from attending the whelping

20.5 INEFFECTUAL STRAINING FOR OVER 1 HOUR

NB: the first pup may live for 6 hours after the onset of straining; subsequent pups usually die if they are not delivered after 2 hours of straining

Possible causes

Reasons for pup not entering the bony pelvis/vagina

❑ pup too large (especially in small litter)
❑ fetal monster, e.g. hydrocephalus, anasarca
❑ transverse presentation, i.e. pup partly in both uterine horns; it cannot then enter the uterine body
❑ ventral flexion of the nose so that the poll of the head engages the pelvic inlet
❑ lateral deviation of the head and neck; may feel one leg in vagina
❑ complete ventral deviation of head and neck
❑ pup cannot get up to pelvic inlet due to pendulous abdomen, e.g. in boxers
❑ dead pup

Pup in vagina, but progressing slowly

❑ relatively large pup

- ☐ posterior presentation of first pup
- ☐ straining not intense enough

Blockage in the vagina

- ☐ tumour (polyp)
- ☐ exostosis or pelvic bone malalignment following a previous fracture
- ☐ congenital vaginal stenosis, usually due to a longitudinal band of tissue which runs the length of the vagina; presumably such bitches become pregnant without a 'tie' (see 8.3 and 14.3)

Investigation

Possible findings from digital exploration of the vagina

- ☐ vagina relaxed and moist but no pup present; manipulating a pup in the caudal abdomen with the other hand may make palpation easier
- ☐ fluid filled amnion in vagina
- ☐ part of a pup in the vagina
- ☐ vaginal occlusion due to a polyp, exostosis or stenosis

NB: remember it is not possible to palpate the cranial vagina or cervix digitally because of its length

Radiology or ultrasonography

- ☐ this is to assess the viability and number of pups

Treatment

- ☐ if nothing felt in vagina – caesarean operation
- ☐ if amnion only felt – lift fetus transabdominally with other hand and stimulate the dorsal wall of the vagina to cause contractions
- ☐ if vaginal occlusion – caesarean operation
- ☐ if fetal malposition – see obstetrical manipulation (20.8)

20.6 BITCH HAD SEVERAL PUPPIES BUT RESTLESS OR LARGER LITTER EXPECTED

Possible causes

- ☐ pup in cranial vagina resulting in no further contractions
- ☐ secondary uterine inertia
- ☐ normal rest between puppies
- ☐ no more pups present

Investigation

- ☐ digital exploration *per vaginam*

❏ palpation; the involuting uterus can feel quite turgid and should not be mistaken for another pup
❏ radiography; the presence or absence of fetal bones
❏ ultrasonography; the involuting uterus has a characteristic appearance. There is normally a central echogenic region with pools of heterogenous fluid

Treatment

❏ if pups present and no discharge – oxytocin administration
❏ if discharge suggesting placental breakdown and more than one pup left – consider caesarean operation

20.7 OXYTOCIN TREATMENT

❏ oxytocin causes rhythmic uterine contractions
❏ its half life is short, but it can cause powerful contractions
❏ small doses, e.g. 2–4 IU, should be administered initially; if no effect is seen after 10–20 minutes, the same or a larger dose may be given
❏ if delivery of a pup is stimulated by oxytocin, administration may be necessary for subsequent pups
❏ where many pups are still to be born, the use of caesarean operation should be considered
❏ oxytocin should *not* be given in obstructive dystocia or if the cervix is not thought to be relaxed (this requires endoscopic inspection)

20.8 OBSTETRICAL MANIPULATION

❏ this may be done with fingers, vectis or whelping forceps
❏ a clean strong teaspoon may be used like a vectis
❏ ensure asepsis as far as is possible
❏ for finger manipulations it may be possible to push the pup caudally using transabdominal manipulation with the other hand
❏ most live pups make sucking movements when a finger is put in their mouths
❏ the pup's head or hips may be gripped between the crooked index and second fingers
❏ flexed front legs and back legs (breech) may be reached by passing the index finger transversely over the dorsum (shoulder or pelvis) of the pup and flicking the limb backwards; the procedure is repeated with the other hand in bilateral flexions
❏ a vectis and finger are probably preferable to forceps
❏ forceps should be used gently to avoid:
  (a) vaginal damage
  (b) compression of the fetus, particularly the skull
  (c) amputation of extremities
❏ drying of the vagina should be avoided by using a water soluble lubricant

❑ if a pup appears to be 'stuck', slight rotation may assist delivery
❑ traction should be applied if possible whilst the bitch is straining
❑ pressure on the vaginal roof with the fingers may stimulate straining
❑ caesarean operation (see 27.1) should be considered if:
   (a) no progress is made after 15 minutes
   (b) the vagina becomes traumatized
   (c) the bitch becomes distressed
   (d) there are many pups yet to be born

NB: the decision to use caesarean operation is often difficult at the time and retrospective analysis is always easy; the responsibility of the clinician is for the comfort and life of the bitch and her pups. It is often quicker and safer to perform a caesarean operation than to embark on obstetrical manipulation, particularly in small bitches; relief of obstructive dystocia is often followed by secondary inertia

20.9 UTERINE RUPTURE

❑ this appears to occur spontaneously in mid pregnancy (see 19.7) or at term
❑ pups are found alive or dead in the abdomen at laparotomy; rupture of the uterus is evident
❑ may cause polydipsia, vomiting, depression and pyrexia
❑ diagnosis before surgery is often difficult
❑ fetuses which have been in the abdomen for some time will be mummified and may remain there for years
❑ extensive abdominal adhesions may result

20.10 UTERINE TORSION

❑ usually occurs in late pregnancy
❑ can occur in the non-pregnant uterus
❑ causes severe abdominal pain and reluctance to move
❑ can only be diagnosed at laparotomy
❑ hysterectomy or hysterotomy may be performed depending upon the viability of the uterus

20.11 RETAINED FETAL MEMBRANES

❑ the condition is uncommon
❑ the placenta is usually passed within 20 minutes of each pup
❑ retention is usually suspected if a green/black discharge persists after parturition; it is usually caused by a remaining pup and membranes
❑ diagnosis is difficult and requires ultrasound examination or clinical experience
❑ in suspected cases, oxytocin and antibiotics should be given
❑ metritis is a common sequal

20.12 POST-PARTUM METRITIS

❑ bacterial invasion of the uterus following parturition, abortion, manipulation or retention
❑ foul smelling red discharge from vulva
❑ bitch toxaemic, depressed, anorexic and producing no milk
❑ pups crying due to cold and hunger
❑ may be associated with retained pup or membranes
❑ temperature raised initially
❑ may be fatal despite treatment

Treatment

❑ metritis is a bacterial infection without an underlying hormonal component, cf. pyometra
❑ antibiotics, e.g. intravenous ampicillin or potentiated sulphonamide
❑ intravenous fluid, e.g. Hartmann's solution
❑ oxytocin or ergometrine to stimulate uterine activity and induce discharge of uterine fluid
❑ low dose prostaglandin therapy may also be used to stimulate myometrial activity
❑ ovariohysterectomy may be considered if a pup is retained
❑ uterine lavage with chlorhexidine via laparotomy has been described

20.13 POST-PARTUM HAEMORRHAGE

❑ usually comes from uterus but may be vagina; often the result of physical injuries
❑ flesh blood clots passed frequently
❑ may be associated with coagulopathy
❑ give oxytocin and antibiotics; expulsion of blood by the former may initially make the condition look worse
❑ ergometrine may be preferable to oxytocin because it provides a prolonged initial contraction of the uterus
❑ blood transfusion and/or ovariohysterectomy may be considered

20.14 SUBINVOLUTION OF PLACENTAL SITES

❑ some degree of vulval discharge is normal for a week or so following whelping
❑ if a serosanguinous discharge persists, it is most probably due to sub-involution of the uterus at one or more of the placental sites; haemorrhage continues from the endometrium at the position of the marginal haematoma (see 11.4)
❑ the bitch shows no signs of malaise
❑ palpation and ultrasonography may reveal discrete areas of uterine enlargement

❏ antibiotics and ecbolic drugs will not help to terminate the condition
❏ recently the combined administration of progestogens and antibiotics was found to be useful in a limited number of cases
❏ usually haemorrhage occurs until the next oestrus, after which it resolves
❏ subsequent fertility is not affected
❏ if bleeding is marked, the bitch should be examined for anaemia
❏ ovariohysterectomy may be necessary if bleeding is severe, although it is very rare for this to be the case

20.15 HYPOCALCAEMIA (PUERPERAL TETANY OR ECLAMPSIA)

❏ most common in small breeds
❏ most common in early lactation but can occur in late pregnancy
❏ clinical signs are nervousness, panting, whining, hypersalivation and a stiff gait
❏ there is frequently a marked pyrexia
❏ if untreated, tonic or clonic muscular spasms may occur
❏ treatment is 5–20 ml 10% calcium borogluconate intravenously slowly; then give the same volume subcutaneously
❏ cardiac rate and rhythm should be monitored during intravenous administration
❏ feed the pups artificially for 24 hours or wean completely
❏ may give bromocriptine or cabergoline (see 24.8) to stop lactation (often causes vomiting)
❏ oral calcium supplementation may be tried in bitches at risk (see inertia) but this may depress parathyroid hormone production and exacerbate the problem if given before whelping

20.16 CANNIBALISM

❏ nervous (often inexperienced) bitches may neglect or kill pups if they are disturbed, particularly by strangers
❏ bitches may neglect individual pups; sometimes they have obvious defects, e.g. small size, cleft palate
❏ excess chewing of the umbilical cord may be extended to eating part of the abdominal wall of the pup
❏ excess licking may cause ulceration of the limbs, etc. of pups

20.17 PROLAPSED UTERUS

❏ very rare
❏ occurs during the periparturient period when the cervix is open
❏ may be incomplete in which case the bitch strains and the prolapse can be palpated in the vagina
❏ repositioning may be possible *per vaginam*

❏   otherwise a laparotomy should be performed to pull the uterus back into the abdomen
❏   amputation has been described
❏   fatal haemorrhage may occur from the uterine vessels

21 Approach to Infertility Cases

21.1 DEFINITIONS

Fertility: capability of producing offspring

Sterility: absolute inability to produce offspring

Infertility: strictly this word is synonymous with sterility; however, it is often used to denote a reduced ability to produce offspring which is below the normal for that species or breed

Subfertility: a less than average ability to produce offspring; sometimes used synonymously with infertility

21.2 EXPECTATIONS OF FERTILITY

- ❏ about 80% of mated bitches produce pups
- ❏ possible litter sizes vary greatly in different breeds
- ❏ neither bitches nor dogs are often exploited for maximal production, so that ideal total pup output cannot be defined
- ❏ in breeding kennels the rate of pup production is usually related to demand, which may be influenced by time of year or other factors
- ❏ for the veterinary surgeon the earliest definition of a fertility problem is when the owner of either dog, bitch or kennels is disappointed by results; often the owner has eliminated some of the possible causes so that questions regarding previous breeding history should be put tactfully
- ❏ in general, advice is sought after a dog has mated three bitches, or a bitch has been mated at two heats, unsuccessfully

21.3 THE INFERTILE BITCH

Infrequent oestrus

- ❏ delayed puberty (see 17.1)
- ❏ long inter-oestrous interval (see 17.5)
- ❏ poor observation by owner

Mating difficulties

- ❏ inexperienced dog (see 8.4)
- ❏ inexperienced bitch (see 8.4)
- ❏ psychological problem in the dog (see 8.4 and 18.6)

❏ psychological problem in the bitch (see 8.4 and 17.10)
❏ bitch not 'ready' (see 8.2)
❏ vulval stenosis (see 14.1)
❏ vestibular constriction (see 14.2)
❏ vaginal constriction (see 14.3)
❏ incompatibility of size: this is rarely a serious problem although failure to mate for other reasons may be blamed onto a size difference
❏ no 'tie' (see 8.4)
❏ vaginal hyperplasia and protrusion (see 14.3)
❏ vaginal tumours (see 14.3)

Failure to conceive after normal mating

❏ mating at wrong time (see 8.2 and 17.6)
❏ mating by infertile dogs
❏ uterine aplasia (see 14.5)
❏ tubal lesions (see 14.6)
❏ vaginal 'infection' is probably not a cause of infertility (see 4.5, 4.10 and 14.3)

Pregnancy failure

❏ resorption (see 19.3)
❏ abortion (see 19.5)

21.4 TREATMENT OF INFERTILITY IN THE BITCH

Delayed puberty and long inter-oestrus

❏ consider oestrus induction (see below)
❏ if this is unsuccessful, consider exploratory laparotomy or laparoscopy to check for the presence of ovaries

Oestrus induction

Oestrogens

❏ low doses of oestrogen enable follicle stimulating hormone (FSH) to stimulate the formation of luteinizing hormone (LH) receptors on granulosa cells and therefore increase the responsiveness to basal concentrations of LH:
(a) the result is follicular growth and production of oestrogen
(b) gonadotrophin concentrations are low due to the negative feedback effect
(c) as follicles mature their walls luteinize and progesterone is produced
(d) the decline in the oestrogen:progesterone ratio facilitates the pre-ovulatory LH surge
❏ the induction of oestrus with diethylstilboestrol has been used clinically for some time

❏ in one study when diethylstilboestrol was administered until 2 days after the onset of pro-oestrus and ovulation was ensured by the administration of FSH and LH all bitches became pregnant and whelped normally
❏ subsequent studies have not, however, been as successful, although more recently diethylstilboestrol alone produced good results

Gonadotrophins

❏ repeated doses of equine chorionic gonadotrophin (eCG) given to anoestrous bitches stimulates follicular growth and the production of oestrogen:
(a) ovulation may occur spontaneously, following an endogenous surge of LH
(b) ovulation may need to be induced using human chorionic gonado-trophin (hCG)
❏ these regimes are more effective in late anoestrous bitches compared with those in early anoestrus
❏ care must be observed when using eCG and hCG combinations because endogenous hyperoestrogenism may occur and result in inhibition of implantation, bone marrow suppression and death
❏ low doses of gonadotrophins are suggested to produce more physiological plasma oestrogen profiles
❏ a relatively low plasma progesterone concentration or short luteal phase following gonadotrophin-induced oestrus is common; this effect might be mediated by the high endogenous or exogenous oestrogen concentration inhibiting release of the luteotrophic gonadotrophin LH

Prolactin antagonists

❏ apparently normal and fertile oestrous periods may be induced in anoes-trous bitches following continual administration of bromocriptine or caber-goline
❏ the time to the onset of oestrus seems to relate to the stage of anoestrus; bitches in late anoestrus respond more quickly than those in early anoestrus
❏ treatment starting in the luteal phase may also be effective, but the treatment period is longer
❏ the induced oestrus appears to be physiological, and whilst the mechanism of action is uncertain it may be the result of inhibition of remnant proges-terone production by the corpora lutea

Inability to mate

❏ ensure that the bitch is properly in oestrus
❏ eliminate physical obstructions as a cause of pain at the time of mating
❏ familiarize the bitch with the mating environment
❏ consider using a different dog that is less (or more) dominant
❏ consider using an anxiolytic or sedative agent
❏ consider artificial insemination

Failure to conceive after normal matings

❑ choose a fertile dog
❑ consider investigating thyroid function
❑ perform a complete pre-breeding investigation including ultrasonography of the uterus to rule out uterine disease such as cystic endometrial hyperplasia
❑ ascertain that mating occurs at the right time at the next oestrus (see Chapter 10)
❑ ensure that bacterial colonization of the uterus does not occur by administering a 6-day course of a broad spectrum antibiotic after mating; it has not been proven that this problem occurs (see 21.7) and the aim is to limit proliferation of commensal organisms
❑ consider exploratory laparotomy to ensure the presence of a normal uterus, oviducts and ovaries
❑ routine bacteriological screening has little role in investigating these cases
NB: since the timing of oestrus and the timing of ovulation during oestrus can be quite erratic in normal bitches, few decisions can be made in the light of the previous breeding history

21.5 THE INFERTILE DOG

Failure to copulate (see 8.4 and 18.6)

❑ inexperience
❑ uncooperative bitch
❑ psychological reasons
❑ physical reasons

Failure of conception after normal matings

❑ failure to ejaculate – this has never been described (see 18.5)
❑ testicular atrophy due to steroids (see 15.3 and 24.1, 24.2, 24.3, 24.10)
❑ spermatogenic arrest (see 15.3)
❑ testicular aplasia (congenital) (see 15.3)
❑ testicular degeneration (see 15.3)
❑ poor semen quality (see 9.5)
❑ mating infertile bitches

21.6 TREATMENT OF INFERTILITY IN THE DOG (see 8.4 and 18.6)

Failure to copulate

❑ eliminate obvious physical reasons
❑ let the dog run with an experienced bitch
❑ try a different bitch

❏ minerals, vitamins and homeopathic remedies have not been shown to be effective but probably do no harm
❏ *do not* give androgens or gonadotrophins as they are not effective and may be detrimental to spermatogenesis (see 24.3 and 24.4)
❏ thyroid replacement therapy may be tried in dogs with musculo-skeletal problems having no hereditary component
❏ try non-steroidal anti-inflammatory agents

Failure to achieve conception

❏ ensure that the dog is mated with a 'proven' bitch
❏ perform breeding soundness examination and collect and evaluate semen quality (see Chapter 9 and 15.3)

Morphological abnormalities (teratozoospermia)

❏ may occur following pyrexia, and resolves quickly (within 60 days) of this event
❏ minor or major abnormalities in semen quality may be the result of drugs or toxins affecting spermatogenesis or the epididymal phase of development. Drugs known to have a deleterious effect include:
(a) androgens
(b) oestrogens
(c) corticosteroids
(d) GnRH agonists and antagonists
(e) ketoconazole
❏ occasionally seen in the early stages of spermatogenic arrest when the principal abnormality relates to thickening of the mid piece
❏ an inherited mid piece defect that develops after 4 years of age has been recognized in certain breeds, e.g. springer spaniels
❏ may occur in the early stages of testicular degeneration secondary to some other pathological process

Abnormalities of spermatozoal number (oligozoospermia)

❏ obstruction of the epididymides or ductus deferens is rare but may be diagnosed by measuring epididymal markers in the ejaculate; there is currently no suitable treatment
❏ may occur in dogs treated with exogenous steroids that have a negative feedback effect upon the hypothalamus and pituitary gland
❏ similarly seen in the early stages of dogs with Sertoli cell tumours that secrete oestrogen
❏ seen in dogs with testicular hypoplasia, although more commonly these are azoospermic
❏ seen in dogs with retrograde ejaculation, although usually no fluid is ejaculated in these cases

Absence of spermatozoa (azoospermia)

❑ seen in the end stage of testicular disease, e.g. following testicular degeneration, autoimmune orchitis, orchitis
❑ found in dogs with testicular hypoplasia
❑ found in dogs with bilateral outflow obstruction
❑ there is no treatment

Abnormalities of spermatozoal motility (asthenozoospermia)

❑ frequently related to abnormal spermatozoal morphology, i.e. mid piece abnormalities
❑ may occasionally be seen in dogs with sperm–sperm agglutination
❑ no suitable treatment has been described

Abnormalities of spermatozoal morphology, number and motility (oligoasthenoteratozoospermia)

❑ may occur during testicular degeneration
❑ observed in many of the above listed pathological processes

21.7 INFERTILITY IN KENNELS

The problem

❑ usually more than one male dog involved
❑ male dogs from outside the kennels (and not known to be infertile) may be involved
❑ rate of pup production is significantly reduced
❑ may be longer than expected interval between successive periods of oestrus
❑ when matings occur, conception rates are lower than previously expected
❑ there may be an increase in the production of dead pups at term
❑ the death rate of pups during the first week (fading pups) may increase
❑ the problem may occur gradually or suddenly in established kennels with previous satisfactory fertility

Possible causes

❑ no cause has ever been proven and in most cases there may be a combination of aetiologies
❑ abortion, stillbirths and fading pups are often associated with infection, but the aetiology is often not proven, despite intensive investigations (see 19.5)
❑ infertility in a well established kennels has been said to be due to the premises becoming 'dog-sick'; in many cases hygiene and management are adequate by currently perceived standards

Possible treatments

- ❑ eliminate the male dog as a cause, i.e. semen evaluation
- ❑ ensure that management factors are adequate; that oestrus is being detected and bitches are mated at the appropriate time
- ❑ oestrus induction may be considered where the inter-oestrus interval is prolonged
- ❑ investigate general hygiene and puppy care, especially in cases of fading puppies
- ❑ when persistent abortion occurs bacteriological/serological investigations of each bitch should be performed to rule out infectious agents (see 19.5)
- ❑ where stillbirths or 'fading pups' are a problem bacteriological and serological investigations should be performed on each bitch
- ❑ moving premises may on some occasions be the only way of restoring fertility to a kennels, but is a last resort and may be costly

21.8 WHY DO WE KNOW SO LITTLE ABOUT INFERTILITY IN DOGS?

Lack of pressure

- ❑ the maximal breeding potential of bitches is rarely exploited due to lack of demand
- ❑ compared with other domesticated animals, low fertility is tolerated
- ❑ because most dogs are not bred for commercial interests, many infertile animals are not investigated
- ❑ dogs are selected for looks or performance, not for fertility
- ❑ usually advice is only sought when the patient is a champion or the 'last of a line'
- ❑ owners are often reluctant to admit to a fertility problem in their dogs because they are worried that others will presume the condition is infectious or inherited

Difficulty of investigation in the bitch

- ❑ knowledge concerning the significance of vaginal bacteria is usually mis-informed (see 4.5 and 14.3)
- ❑ digital examination of the whole vagina is impossible, even in large bitches
- ❑ visual examination of the whole vagina is very difficult (see 4.7)
- ❑ catheterization of the cervix for visualization, swabbing and biopsy of the endometrium is difficult
- ❑ radiography of the vagina and uterus is only possible using contrast media, and information gained from the uterus is not interpretable at the moment
- ❑ ultrasonography of the uterus in the absence of gross distension is confined to the distal body where it passes over the bladder (see 12.9)
- ❑ ultrasonography of the ovaries is very difficult, but is possible during oestrus; few pathological changes have been described and, although the

detection of follicular growth is possible, the diagnosis of ovulation is prevented by the fact that follicles do not collapse at this time (see 1.8)

❑ in order to detect hormone abnormalities, bitches would need to be bled at least twice daily over the period when suspected malfunction was to occur; this is usually impractical and expensive (see Chapter 3)

❑ in order to detect anomalies of pregnancy development, repeated ultrasonographic examinations would be necessary; this would be expensive

Difficulty in investigating the dog

❑ semen collection and identification of dogs with poor semen quality is easy

❑ obtaining stud dogs for further investigation, particularly castration and examination of testicular tissue, is very difficult as owners do not usually wish to donate this material

❑ investigation of possible methods of improving fertility in dogs is difficult because the owners of infertile dogs do not wish them to be used for research

22 Artificial Insemination

Artificial insemination (AI) is the technique of collecting semen from a male animal, and placing it into the reproductive tract of the female.

❏ AI may involve the use of:
   (a) freshly collected semen
   (b) semen that has been diluted and chilled
   (c) semen that has been frozen and thawed
❏ AI is widely used throughout the world
❏ in the UK there is limited use of AI because of the restrictions imposed by the Kennel Club
❏ there is, however, increasing interest in frozen semen inseminations in the UK
❏ before AI is undertaken a semen sample should be collected from the dog to ensure it is of suitable quality, and to familiarize the dog with the procedure

22.1 ADVANTAGES OF ARTIFICIAL INSEMINATION

❏ reduces the requirement to transport animals
❏ overcomes the quarantine restrictions that prevent the movement of animals from one country to another
❏ increases the genetic pool available to an individual breed within a country
❏ reduces the disease risk when unknown animals enter a kennel for mating
❏ in some countries the use of AI may reduce the spread of infectious diseases
❏ in certain circumstances, artificial insemination may be useful when natural mating is difficult, for example bitches which ovulate when they are not in standing oestrus or bitches that have hyperplasia of the vaginal floor
❏ semen may be collected from male animals which due to age, debility, back pain or premature ejaculation are unable to achieve a natural mating
❏ the greatest area of interest is probably the storage of genetic material by freezing semen for insemination at a future date

22.2 DISADVANTAGES OF ARTIFICIAL INSEMINATION

❏ collection of semen from some dogs may be difficult
❏ theoretically a dog could become 'overused' within a population
❏ semen from some dogs is not suitable for chilling or freeze-thawing
❏ there is the potential for error in sample identification

22.3 REGULATIONS CONCERNING THE USE OF ARTIFICIAL INSEMINATION

❏ in the UK, pups which are the result of AI can only be registered if the Kennel Club has given prior permission
❏ other registration organisations have different regulations
❏ in the UK, the permission of the Kennel Club is not required before semen is imported or exported
❏ specific regulations are set by the Ministry of Agriculture Fisheries and Food in the UK regarding semen import
❏ specific regulations are set by countries other than the UK regarding semen import; these vary and should always be checked before embarking on semen transportation

22.4 METHODS OF SEMEN USE

Fresh semen

❏ may be used diluted or undiluted
❏ may be used when there is inability to mate the bitch (aggressive bitch, unwilling dog, injury)

Chilled semen

❏ semen may be stored for a short period of time by chilling and rewarming:
  (a) this allows transportation of semen
  (b) this may be useful when there is short term unavailability of the dog

Frozen semen

❏ semen may be stored for long periods of time by freezing and thawing:
  (a) this allows transportation of semen
  (b) genetic material may be stored for a long period of time

22.5 PATHOGENS THAT MAY BE SPREAD IN DOG SEMEN

❏ little information is known about transmission of infectious organisms in semen:
  (a) canine herpes virus may be transmitted at coitus, but it seems likely that this is via direct contact rather than within semen
  (b) rabies virus is unlikely to be found in semen except possibly during a few days before overt clinical signs of the disease
  (c) canine transmissible venereal tumour may be transmitted at coitus, probably by contact and not in semen

22.6 SEMEN PRESERVATION

❏ semen may be preserved by the following methods:
  (a) fresh and cooled to room temperature

(b) diluted and cooled to 5°C

(c) diluted and frozen (–196°C) then thawed

❏ the lifespan of preserved semen depends upon the preservation method:

(a) fresh semen: 4 hours (although this may be extended by initial dilution)

(b) diluted and cooled semen: 4 days

(c) diluted and frozen semen: indefinite

❏ semen is normally diluted in an 'extender solution' which aims to:

(a) protect spermatozoa during cooling/freezing/warming

(b) supply an energy source to spermatozoa

(c) maintain pH, osmolarity and ionic strength

❏ for many species the optimal pH for survival is approximately 7.0. During storage hydrogen ions are produced by spermatozoa therefore the pH falls. Control of pH is important and many agents have been used:

(a) phosphate buffer

(b) egg yolk

(c) milk proteins

(d) zwitterionic buffers, e.g. Tris, Tes, Hepes

❏ hypotonic diluents are harmful because they lead to a gain in intracellular water and redistribution of ions; hypertonic diluents are less harmful because they lead to water loss and a reduction in the likelihood of intracellular ice crystallization. Seminal plasma is 300 mOsm; thus most diluents are approximately 370 mOsm

❏ glucose, fructose and mannose are glycolysable sugars that may be included in semen extenders as sources of energy

❏ the larger molecular weight sugars (ribose, arabinose) are often used as non-penetrating cryoproctectants

❏ antibacterial agents are usually included in semen extenders to control proliferation of microorganisms

❏ specific protective agents may be used including:

(a) milk proteins which protect against cold shock

(b) egg yolk (low density lipoproteins) and bovine serum albumen which protect acrosomal and mitochondrial membranes, and protect against cold shock

❏ cryoprotective agents are essential for semen freezing because they prevent ice crystal damage; they may be divided into those that are:

(a) penetrating, (e.g. glycerol and dimethyl sulphoxide (DMSO))

(b) non-penetrating, (e.g. sugars and polyvinyl pyrollidone)

22.7 PREPARATION OF FRESH DOG SEMEN

❏ a semen sample is collected as previously described (see 9.5)

❏ the second fraction is evaluated and used for insemination

❏ one ejaculate is used for each insemination

❏ once collected, semen may be deposited into the vagina of the bitch using a long inseminating pipette which is gently introduced near to the cervix (see 1.5)

❏ when semen is placed in this position spermatozoa must swim through the cervix, into the uterus and up the uterine horns

❏ vaginal insemination is not ideal, but with good quality fresh semen provides reasonable success

22.8 PREPARATION OF CHILLED DOG SEMEN

❏ a common extender is composed of non-fat dry milk (e.g. Marvel), 2.4 g; glucose, 4.9 g; sodium bicarbonate, 0.15 g; sufficient deionized water to make the volume up to 100 ml. Antimicrobial agents may then be added: penicillin 150 000 IU, and streptomycin 150 000 mg

❏ alternatively a low fat pasteurized cow's milk extender can be prepared by heating the milk until it starts to simmer, and then allowing it to cool to 37°C

❏ the extender is kept at 37°C in a water bath immediately before use

❏ the semen is collected and evaluated

❏ a small portion of semen is mixed with a small volume of the extender and then evaluated

❏ providing that the extender has no deleterious effect, the remaining semen is diluted with the extender at 37°C

❏ it is preferable to dilute the semen in a semen:extender ratio of 1:4

❏ the extended semen is cooled slowly to 5°C and stored at this temperature

❏ slow cooling can be achieved by placing the extended semen in an insulated vial which is then put in a refrigerator

❏ semen may be transported before being inseminated

❏ transportation can be easily achieved using a wide mouthed thermos flask partially filled with ice cubes

❏ it is important to perform a trial storage before shipping semen

❏ semen is normally warmed slowly by placing the vials in a water bath at 37°C

22.9 PREPARATION OF FROZEN–THAWED DOG SEMEN

❏ an extender containing: Tris, 6.06 g; fructose, 2.5 g; citric acid, 3.4 g; deionized water, 184 ml is used. To this is added glycerol and egg yolk to a final concentration of 8% and 20%, respectively. Often penicillin and streptomycin are added to the extender before use as described above

❏ a small portion of semen is mixed with a small volume of the extender and then evaluated

❏ providing that the extender has no deleterious effect, the remaining semen is diluted with the extender at 37°C:

(a) it is preferable to make a volume:volume dilution rather than to try and obtain a standard spermatozoal concentration

(b) the optimal dilution rate appears to be 1:4 (semen:extender)

❏ following dilution the sample is re-evaluated, and then placed in insulated vials

❏ vials are slowly cooled to 5°C and allowed to equilibrate for 2–4 hours

❑ diluted semen is then loaded into 0.5 ml straws in a cold room
❑ straws are frozen at standard freezing rates in liquid nitrogen vapour, before being plunged into liquid nitrogen
❑ straws are generally thawed rapidly (70°C for 10 seconds) before being placed at 37°C

22.10 INSEMINATION

❑ the accurate timing of insemination is essential when poor quality semen is used, or when the use of cryopreserved semen is contemplated (this has short longevity in the female tract):
(a) the ideal time is between 2 and 5 days after ovulation
(b) for frozen semen, insemination should be performed on the basis of plasma (serum) progesterone (or LH) measurement (detection of the fertilization period) (see 10.1)
(c) for chilled semen, insemination should be performed on the basis of plasma (serum) progesterone (or LH) measurement
(d) for fresh semen, insemination may be performed on the basis of vaginal endoscopy and vaginal cytological assessment (detection of the fertile period)
❑ a minimum of 200×10^6 normal motile spermatozoa should be present in each inseminate
❑ natural mating results in vaginal contractions that propel the ejaculate cranially into the uterus; these contractions are generally absent when a bitch is artificially inseminated and therefore spermatozoal transport is reduced
❑ uterine insemination results in a higher success rate than does vaginal insemination:
(a) for reasonable success with frozen semen uterine insemination is necessary
(b) vaginal insemination may give reasonable success with fresh semen

22.11 INSEMINATION TECHNIQUES

Intravaginal insemination

❑ a rigid plastic catheter is required, about 30 cm long for a large bitch
❑ attach a plastic syringe; if this has a rubber plunger it is best to wash the syringe out first with distilled water as rubber is toxic to spermatozoa
❑ suck the inseminate into the catheter; if fresh semen is being used (small volume) it need not enter the syringe
❑ initially the catheter is introduced vertically through the vulval lips, but at the level of the ischium it is directed cranially; the vagina of the bitch is relatively long (see 1.4)
❑ if the bitch will allow, the catheter can usually be palpated through the abdominal wall and the cervix is located as a hard structure cranial to it
❑ the bitch's hind limbs are raised off the ground and the semen expelled; it

may then be necessary to inject air down the catheter to ensure that it is empty
- ❑ stimulating the bitch's vestibule with a finger is said to stimulate vaginal contractions which aid passage of semen into the uterus
- ❑ after about 10 minutes, or if the bitch struggles violently, she is allowed to stand
- ❑ urination should be prevented for 10 minutes; reflux of a lot of fluid indicates a poor insemination
- ❑ the timing of insemination is discussed in 8.2; two inseminations should be made where possible, on alternate days

Intrauterine insemination

- ❑ it is very difficult to place a catheter through the bitch's cervix into the uterus because:
  - (a) the vagina is long and narrow (up to 20 cm long)
  - (b) the cervical opening is small, and placed at an angle to the vagina
- ❑ several methods have therefore been developed to allow uterine insemination

Foley catheter technique

- ❑ manufactured by IMV in France
- ❑ an especially designed Foley catheter may be used to perform an effective uterine insemination:
  - (a) the catheter has the bulb positioned at the catheter tip
  - (b) a second catheter with a side exit port is inserted through the Foley catheter
- ❑ the catheter is inserted into the vagina up to the level of the cervix and the bulb is inflated; this forms a seal against the cranial vaginal wall
- ❑ the second catheter is advanced and the semen is deposited; semen can only run forwards through the cervix and does not drain back along the vagina
- ❑ the second catheter is withdrawn inside the Foley catheter, thereby closing the side exit ports
- ❑ both catheters are left in place for up to 15 minutes:
  - (a) this ensures that a pool of semen is located next to the cervix
  - (b) this may simulate the copulatory tie and result in vaginal contractions
- ❑ the principle of the technique is excellent, but there is often leakage of semen around, and through the catheters

Norwegian catheter technique

- ❑ available from Dr. J. Fougner in Norway (Fig. 22.1)
- ❑ consists of an outer plastic catheter and inner metal catheter with rounded bulb-ended tip
- ❑ the outer plastic catheter is inserted into the vagina to the level of the cervix
- ❑ the cervix is palpated transabdominally

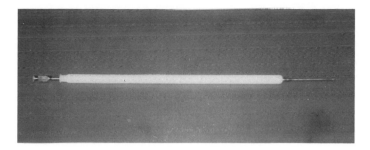

Fig. 22.1 Norwegian catheter: a white coloured soft plastic outer catheter and inner metal catheter with round-bulbed end.

❏ the inner catheter is pushed forwards to the cervix and at the same time the cervix is reorientated transabdominally; the aim is to produce a straight line from the vagina into the cervix so that the inner catheter can be directed through the cervical canal
❏ this technique works very well but requires training and considerable practice
❏ it is impossible in large, obese or frightened animals with a tense abdomen

Endoscopic technique

❏ this method requires a rigid endoscope and inflation system, preferably with a mechanism for deflecting a catheter at the endoscope tip (Fig. 22.2)
❏ the endoscope is inserted into the vagina and advanced to the level of the cervix
❏ inflation of the vagina is useful for allowing the identification of the cervical os
❏ the os is positioned in the dorsal wall of the vagina
❏ the inseminating catheter is inserted through the endoscope and the deflection device is used to direct the catheter into the os
❏ the technique works very well, although some bitches need to be sedated otherwise movement of the bitch makes placement of the catheter very

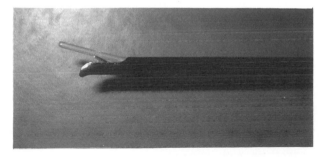

Fig. 22.2 Endoscope with deflection device for direction of an inseminating catheter through the cervical os.

difficult; reversible sedation with the alpha$_2$ adrenoceptor agonist drugs such as medetomidine appears to be ideal
❑ the technique requires training and practice before catheterization can be achieved reliably

Surgical technique

❑ requires general anaesthesia
❑ a small caudal ventral midline laparotomy incision is made
❑ the uterine body is lifted into the incision
❑ a fine over-the-needle intravenous catheter is placed into the lumen of the uterine body
❑ padded bowel clamps are placed on the uterus distal to the catheter
❑ the semen is introduced slowly into the uterus and runs forwards into the uterine horns
❑ following removal of the catheter pressure is applied to the site to provide haemostasis; no sutures are required
❑ the incision is closed routinely
❑ the technique is simple and can be performed rapidly; consideration should, however, be given to the ethics of performing a surgical procedure

22.12 SUCCESS WITH ARTIFICIAL INSEMINATION

❑ spermatozoal longevity is greatest for fresh semen, and least for frozen–thawed semen
❑ fertility rates are related to spermatozoal damage during preservation and to spermatozoal longevity
❑ extensive bitch management is required when frozen–thawed semen is used, since insemination has to be performed during the fertilization period
❑ it may be extremely difficult to preserve the semen from certain dogs; the reason for this is not known
❑ as a guide 'world average' success rates for bitches inseminated at the appropriate time are:
(a) fresh semen: 60–90% pregnancy rate
(b) chilled semen: 50–70% pregnancy rate
(c) frozen semen: 30–60% pregnancy rate
NB: in certain laboratories values may be higher than those above, especially when the semen collection and insemination is performed entirely in-house

23 Hormonal Contraception in the Bitch

❏ unwanted pets are a major social and sometimes ecological problem. They may result in zoonotic disease, pollution and damage to public areas, livestock and man. Millions of unwanted pets are destroyed each year
❏ see chapter 24 for adverse effects of exogenous hormones

23.1 ADVANTAGE OF PREVENTION AND SUPPRESSION OF OESTRUS

❏ abolishes signs of oestrus and the inconvenience they can cause (see 25.1)
❏ prevents pregnancy
❏ usually prevents false pregnancy
❏ is not permanent, i.e. the bitch can be bred from afterwards
❏ NB: chlorophyllin given orally may reduce the sexual attractiveness of some bitches

23.2 DISADVANTAGE OF PREVENTION AND SUPPRESSION OF OESTRUS

❏ requires regular injections or administration of tablets
❏ when used for long periods progestogens can cause side-effects, particularly on the uterus (see 24.1)
❏ is not a substitute for surgical neutering
❏ not recommended for suppression of the first oestrus
❏ some progestogens, e.g. medroxyprogesterone acetate, may cause mammary neoplasia

23.3 SUPPRESSION OF A PRO-OESTRUS THAT HAS ALREADY STARTED

Inject a long-acting progestogen

❏ for example, proligestone
❏ inject *early* in pro-oestrus
NB: progesterone is too rapidly metabolized for this purpose, even when suspended in oil
❏ the bitch sometimes shows discomfort after subcutaneous injection
❏ occasionally an area of alopecia develops over the injection site; for this reason the manufacturers recommend injections on the medial aspect of the flank-fold in show dogs
❏ signs of pro-oestrus usually disappear within 5 days of administration

❑ if given late in pro-oestrus, may predispose to pyometra due to increased progestogenic influence on the uterus when bacteria may be present (cervix relaxed)
❑ the next oestrus can be expected 3–9 (average 6) months later

Administer an 8-day course of an orally active progestogen

❑ for example, megestrol acetate
❑ must start *early* in pro-oestrus
❑ signs of pro-oestrus usually disappear within 2–3 days after the start of the course
❑ if given late in pro-oestrus it is theoretically less likely than a long-acting progestogen to predispose to pyometra because the course of drug administration is short
❑ oestrus may recur any time after 4 months later

23.4 PREVENTION OF AN EXPECTED PRO-OESTRUS/OESTRUS

❑ sometimes an expected oestrus is likely to coincide with a social or another event which makes management of the oestrous bitch difficult
❑ treatment should be given in anoestrus, i.e. more than 2 months after the end of the previous oestrus; because the length of anoestrus is very long and variable in the bitch, the timing of the treatment is governed by the time when oestrus is to be avoided

Subcutaneous administration of depot preparations during anoestrus

❑ depot progestogens (medroxyprogesterone acetate, delmadinone acetate, and proligestone) administered during anoestrus will prevent a subsequent oestrus
❑ medroxyprogesterone acetate and proligestone are licensed for this purpose in the bitch

Oral administration of progestogens during anoestrus

❑ low doses of orally active progestogens (megestrol acetate, medroxyprogesterone acetate, norethisterone acetate) can be used to prevent oestrus for as long as administration is continued
❑ megestrol acetate and medroxyprogesterone acetate are licensed for this purpose in the bitch
❑ should the animal enter proestrus during the first few days of treatment, the dosage can be increased
❑ a period of anoestrus usually follows therapy so oestrus does not return immediately after cessation of treatment

Oral administration of synthetic androgens during anoestrus

❏ a synthetic androgen mibolerone, which is not available in the UK is effective for the prevention of oestrus in bitches
❏ mibolerone is formulated as a liquid for daily oral administration
❏ mibolerone has adverse effects typical of other androgens, including clitoral hypertrophy, vaginitis, and behavioural changes; in addition, anal gland abnormalities, obnoxious body odour and obesity have also been recorded

Administration of depot androgens during anoestrus

❏ administration of testosterone either as a prolonged release implant, or depot injection of mixed testosterone esters may be used to prevent oestrus in bitches

23.5 PREVENTION OF REPRODUCTIVE BEHAVIOUR FOR EXTENDED PERIODS OF TIME

It may be convenient to prevent reproductive behaviour for a long period of time when the ultimate aim is still to breed from the bitch

Subcutaneous administration of depot preparations during anoestrus

❏ medroxyprogesterone acetate and proligestone are licensed for this purpose in the bitch
❏ they are normally given at 3, 4 and thereafter 5 month intervals for proligestone, and 6 month intervals for medroxyprogesterone acetate
❏ it may be inadvisable to prevent oestrus for more than 2 years, but providing that a breakthrough cycle does not occur, prolonged prevention may have few adverse effects, especially when using the more recently developed progestogens (proligestone); it has been reported that incidence of pyometra and mammary tumours is reduced compared with untreated females
❏ when therapy is ceased most females cycle normally, although progestogens may induce cystic endometrial hyperplasia and therefore reduce fertility

Short courses of orally active progestogen

❏ for example, megestrol acetate courses are given at the beginning of each pro-oestrus (23.3)
❏ the advantage of such treatment is that progestogen is only given for short periods of time; in some bitches this may be as infrequently as every 8–12 months
❏ the disadvantages are that signs of pro-oestrus must be looked for, and the inconvenience of a few days of pro-oestrus must be endured
❏ other possible side-effects are discussed in 24.1
❏ a period of anoestrus usually follows therapy so oestrus does not return immediately after cessation of treatment

Oral or depot administration of androgens during anoestrus

❏ mibolerone is effective for the long term prevention of oestrus in bitches
❏ often depot androgen therapy (e.g. mixed testosterone esters) is supplemented by daily oral therapy, e.g. testosterone esters are given intramuscularly every 4–6 weeks, with supplemental daily oral testosterone
❏ adverse effects are more common with prolonged therapy
❏ androgens are given at regular intervals to greyhound bitches to prevent oestrus because:
   (a) bitches in oestrus cannot race because they would attract male dogs
   (b) bitches in early metoestrus, i.e. for 10 weeks after the beginning of pro-oestrus, should not race because the high circulating concentrations of progesterone at this time depress performance and make racing predictability difficult
❏ the possible anabolic effects of these preparations appear not to be marked enough to enhance racing performance
❏ there are no known untoward effects on subsequent fertility (see 24.3)
❏ drugs must not be administered to greyhounds during the 7 days before racing

23.6 FUTURE METHODS OF PREVENTING OESTRUS

Gonadotrophin releasing hormone (GnRH) antagonists

❏ GnRH antagonists (e.g. detirelix) have been used to prevent cyclical activity in the bitch
❏ these agents have an immediate onset of action, and may be administered during pro-oestrus:
   (a) they produce a reduction in circulating gonadotrophins within a few hours
   (b) bitches therefore rapidly return to anoestrus
❏ to date, however, their continuous use has potent mast cell degranulating actions

Gonadotrophin releasing hormone agonists

❏ GnRH produces stimulation and then down regulation of GnRH receptors
❏ agonist analogues of GnRH, such as nafarelin, may therefore be used to prevent reproductive cyclicity
❏ most recently, subcutaneously implanted sialastic devices have been used to provide a sustained release of GnRH for up to one year; upon withdrawal bitches returned to cyclical activity within approximately 2 months
❏ these agents are not commercially available

Immunization

❏ immunization of bitches against zona pellucida proteins, gonadotrophins and GnRH may provide an effective means of contraception

❏ a reliable GnRH protein conjugate antigen has recently been developed
❏ such methods require further investigation before they become clinically useful

23.7 UNWANTED MATING

Definitions

Misalliance: is defined in man as an unsuitable marriage

Mesalliance: is defined as an unsuitable marriage between two people of different social backgrounds
NB: in dogs either term is used to describe an unwanted or unplanned mating

The clinical problem

❏ typically the bitch is presented with a history of:
 (a) having been caught 'tied' with a dog (see 8.3)
 (b) having been 'seen' with a male dog
 (c) having escaped for some time and perhaps returned with saliva on her neck, etc.
❏ *therefore* in many cases it is not known whether mating has occurred or not

Examination of the bitch following presumed unwanted mating

❏ the 'blind' treatment of all bitches presumed to have had an unwanted mating may, in certain circumstances, be appropriate
❏ a more satisfactory approach is the careful examination of bitches and the application of treatment in appropriate cases
❏ clinical evaluation of the bitch should involve:
 (a) the collection of a vaginal smear to evaluate the stage of the oestrous cycle and to try to detect spermatozoa
 (b) the use of a modified vaginal smear technique to detect spermatozoa
 (c) the measurement of plasma concentration of progesterone to establish accurately the stage of the oestrous cycle

Vaginal cytology

❏ collection and study of exfoliative vaginal cells may determine the stage of the oestrous cycle (see 4.5)
❏ these results should be used in combination with measurement of plasma concentration of progesterone
❏ in recently mated bitches, spermatozoa may be identified within the vaginal smear
❏ there is however a rapid reduction in the number of spermatozoa and they may not be identified if the interval from mating exceeds 24 hours

Bitches that are found to be in cytological pro-oestrus

❑ in these cases plasma progesterone concentrations are low
❑ such bitches may not have been mated, since mating is usually refused at this time, and therefore do not warrant treatment
❑ however, this is not always the case, and some early matings may result in a pregnancy if the spermatozoa are able to remain viable within the female reproductive tract until after ovulation
❑ assessment of the presence or absence of spermatozoa is therefore essential in these cases

Bitches that are found to be in cytological oestrus

❑ in these cases plasma progesterone concentration is usually intermediate or high
❑ such bitches may have been mated, and in most cases should receive treatment
❑ reference to the presence or absence of spermatozoa may influence whether treatment is instituted

Bitches that are found to be in cytological metoestrus (dioestrus)

❑ in these cases plasma progesterone concentration is high
❑ such bitches may have been mated and should be examined for the presence of spermatozoa
❑ the most important factor is, however, the time interval from mating to examination, because it is rare for matings occurring after the onset of cytological metoestrus (dioestrus) to be fertile

Plasma progesterone measurement

❑ plasma concentrations of progesterone can be measured by ELISA techniques (see 4.9)
   (a) concentrations are low during anoestrus and pro-oestrus
   (b) concentrations increase when pre-ovulatory follicular luteinization occurs
   (c) there is a rapid rise in progesterone concentration after ovulation
❑ progesterone concentrations should be interpreted in the light of the clinical history and assessment of vaginal cytology

Detection of spermatozoa within the vagina

❑ from 24 hours after mating there are few spermatozoa within the vagina
❑ accurate detection of spermatozoa requires a modified cytology technique
❑ a saline-moistened swab should be placed into the vagina for 1 minute
❑ after removal the swab tip should be placed in a small test tube with 0.5 ml physiological saline, and allowed to stand for 10 minutes

❏ the swab is then squeezed dry, and the test tube containing the saline is centrifuged at 2000 rev/min for 10 minutes
❏ collection of the sediment and microscopic examination after staining with a modified Wright–Giemsa stain allows detection of spermatozoal heads
❏ using this technique, spermatozoa are found in 100% of samples in which mating occurred within the previous 24 hours, and in 75% of samples in which mating occurred within the previous 48 hours

Treatment options

❏ there are several treatment options, even when mating has occurred at a time likely to result in conception:
(a) if the bitch is not required for breeding ovariohysterectomy should be performed after the end of oestrus
(b) the bitch may be treated in an attempt to prevent implantation
(c) wait until a positive diagnosis of pregnancy can be made before instituting therapy (requires examination of the bitch at approximately 28 days after mating – see Chapter 12). If a pregnancy is identified it may be terminated by inducing resorption or abortion
❏ treatment options can be considered with respect to the risk of conception (Table 23.1)

Table 23.1 Risk of conception in bitches presumed to have been mated.

Spermatozoa present in vagina	Plasma progesterone concentration	Vaginal cytology examination	Risk of conception
No	Low	Pro-oestrus	Low
No	Low	Oestrus	Low
No	Intermediate/high	Oestrus	Intermediate
No	High	Metoestrus	Low
Yes	Low	Pro-oestrus	Low
Yes	Low	Oestrus	Intermediate
Yes	Intermediate/high	Oestrus	High
Yes	High	Metoestrus	Low

Prevention of implantation

Oestrogens

❏ oestrogens are thought to have several effects that prevent implantation:
(a) they may alter the transport time of zygotes
(b) they may impair implantation
(c) they may cause luteolysis by an uncertain mechanism
(d) they may stimulate uterine contractions and cervical relaxation
❏ diethylstilboestrol injection was used extensively and apparently successfully in the UK until recently; it is no longer available

❑ a course of oral diethylstilboestrol is used in some countries but has not found favour in the UK

❑ oestradiol injection (intramuscularly or subcutaneously) is the treatment of choice; a single injection is given within 4 days after mating

❑ more recently a low dose oestrogen regime at 3 and 5 (and also possibly 7) days after mating, has been introduced

❑ oral ethinyl oestradiol may be effective, but it is not clear whether this drug is active when given by this route in the dog

❑ much of the information on oestrogen treatment in bitches appears to be anecdotal

❑ little scientific interest has been taken into the mode of action of the oestrogens, the optimal dose rate and time of treatment to prevent conception, and the rate of success

❑ clinically, oestrogen seems to be effective at preventing conception, but:
(a) many bitches that are treated were probably not mated
(b) some bitches may have been mated at a time when conception could not occur

❑ possible reasons for treatment failure:
(a) *earlier mating:* than was originally thought, so that treatment is too late
(b) *the shorter half life of oestradiol* compared with diethylstilboestrol, may in some cases allow its effects to have worn off by the time that ova enter the Fallopian trubes; dog sperm can probably remain fertile for up to 7 days in the bitch genital tract (see 8.2)
(c) *the bitch may be mated again after treatment:* in most cases, if the oestradiol is given around the ovulation period, this will not matter because even though oestrus may be prolonged, no new ovulations will be stimulated; if, however, a bitch is treated in pro-oestrus, the drug may have been metabolized by the time of second mating and ovulation

❑ second matings should, however, be discouraged in treated dogs as these may introduce bacteria into the uterus and predispose to pyometra

❑ repeat injections during the same heat should be discouraged as these probably increase the chances of side-effects (see 24.2)

NB: it may be that giving repeated small doses of oestradiol will be more effective and less toxic than giving a single large dose

❑ adverse effects of oestrogens:
(a) oestrogens may potentiate the stimulatory effects of progesterone on the uterus producing cystic endometrial hyperplasia
(b) oestrogens cause cervical relaxation, thus allowing vaginal bacteria to enter the uterus
(c) these two events may result in the development of pyometra
(d) oestrogens also produce dose-related bone marrow suppression
(e) other effects include alopecia, skin hyperpigmentation and mammary and vulval enlargement

Tamoxifen

❑ tamoxifen is an anti-oestrogen which can be used to prevent or terminate pregnancy in the bitch
❑ the exact mechanism of action is unknown; it may interfere with zygote transport and/or implantation
❑ relatively high doses of the drug given twice daily orally during pro-oestrus, oestrus, or early dioestrus are efficacious
❑ a high incidence of pathological changes of the bitch's reproductive tract is induced by tamoxifen, including ovarian cysts and endometritis

Termination of pregnancy

❑ once pregnancy has become established it may be terminated either by altering the endocrine environment or by direct effects upon the embryo
❑ the bitch is dependent upon the ovarian production of progesterone throughout gestation
❑ methods which produce premature luteolysis may therefore be used to terminate pregnancy
❑ both luteinizing hormone (LH) and prolactin have luteotrophic actions; therapy may also be directed against these hormones to cause lysis of the corpora lutea and the termination of pregnancy

Prostaglandins

❑ prostaglandins lyse the corpora lutea and reduce the plasma concentration of progesterone
❑ the corpora lutea of the bitch are more resistant to prostaglandins than other species; repeated therapy is necessary to achieve lysis
❑ prostaglandins also produce contraction of smooth muscle:
   (a) the ecbolic effect may be part of the mechanism of inducing abortion
   (b) however, actions on smooth muscle also account for the adverse effects of prostaglandins including salivation, vomiting, pyrexia, hyperpnoea, ataxia and diarrhoea; high doses may be lethal
❑ pharmacological doses of prostaglandin $F_{2\alpha}$ can be used to produce luteal regression because the duration of treatment is more important than the dose:
   (a) repeated low doses of prostaglandin will significantly reduce plasma progesterone concentration and induce abortion, especially when given later than 25 days after the LH surge
❑ recent studies have, however, shown that daily treatment commencing 5 days after the onset of metoestrus (dioestrus) using high doses of prostaglandin may be efficacious
❑ cloprostenol can also be used to produce abortion 25 days after the LH surge

Prolactin antagonists

❑ bromocriptine and cabergoline reduce plasma concentration of progesterone, especially when administered during the late luteal phase

❏ these agents are dopamine agonists which inhibit the release of prolactin from the anterior pituitary gland
❏ bromocriptine is the least specific agent and tends to produce the most adverse effects, especially vomiting
❏ bromocriptine is, however, the only product available in the UK
❏ when administered during mid-pregnancy both agents produce a significant reduction in plasma progesterone concentration, resulting in resorption or abortion; earlier treatment is less efficacious

Combination of prostaglandin and prolactin antagonists

❏ the combination of the dopamine agonist cabergoline and the synthetic prostaglandin cloprostenol, induces pregnancy termination from day 25 after the LH surge
❏ cabergoline can be administered orally daily, and cloprostenol sub-cutaneously every other day
❏ this regime reduces the adverse effects of prostaglandin therapy alone, and increases the efficacy of prolactin antagonists.
❏ when bitches are treated for approximately 9 days, 100% will resorb, and there are generally no adverse effects

Progesterone antagonists

❏ mifepristone (RU486) and aglepristone (RU534) are progesterone and glucocorticoid receptor antagonists
❏ administration produces an antiprogestogenic effect
❏ when administered to pregnant bitches later than 30 days from the LH surge, fetal death occurs within 5 days of treatment
❏ earlier administration requires a longer treatment period
❏ pregnancy loss is characterized by resorption during early pregnancy or abortion during late pregnancy
❏ adverse effects have not been noted with this treatment
❏ RU534 has recently been marketed for use in bitches in France

Progesterone synthesis inhibitors

❏ epostane is a hydroxysteroid dehydrogenase isomerase enzyme inhibitor which prevents the conversion of pregnenolone to progesterone
❏ a single subcutaneous injection of epostane at the onset of metoestrus (dioestrus) will prevent or terminate pregnancy
❏ injection site abscessation is common
❏ high doses given orally for 7 days will successfully terminate pregnancy without apparent adverse effects
❏ epostane is not available in the UK

Gonadotrophin releasing hormone agonists and antagonists

❏ continous administration of gonadotrophin releasing hormone (GnRH), or

GnRH agonists causes a down-regulation effect which may be used to withdraw gonadotrophin support of the corpus luteum
❏ this produces a decline in progesterone concentration and abortion or resorption
❏ similarly, the daily administration of GnRII *antagonists* successfully suppresses luteal function
❏ these agents are as yet unavailable for this purpose

Corticosteroids

❏ in many species glucocorticoid administration during pregnancy induces abortion
❏ in the bitch repeated administration and high doses are required
❏ the method is impractical and risks adverse effects

Non-hormonal embryotoxic agents
❏ several novel embryotoxic agents have been evaluated in the bitch
❏ lotrifen has a slow release from depot injection and may be efficacious when administered any time during the first 15 days after mating
❏ lotrifen is not available, possibly because of the high incidence of adverse effects which include vomiting, diarrhoea and weight loss

Complications of induced abortion

❏ inconvenience of the haemorrhagic discharge which would accompany placental detachment; the bitch should therefore be hospitalized; ultrasonography (see 12.9) would help in monitoring such cases
❏ uncertainty of knowing whether all fetuses have been aborted or not

24 Pharmacological Control of Reproduction in the Dog and Bitch

24.1 PROGESTOGENS

- ❏ progesterone is produced by the corpora lutea of the bitch, and is not naturally produced by the dog
- ❏ endogenous progesterone suppresses spontaneous myometrial activity and stimulates endometrial growth
- ❏ progesterone is responsible for mammary gland development during the luteal phase
- ❏ progesterone has a feedback effect upon the hypothalamus and pituitary gland
- ❏ progestogens are compounds with progesterone-like activity, and therefore they each exhibit the actions above:

  (a) it is, however, their negative feedback effect upon the hypothalamus and pituitary gland that is the principal reason why they are so widely used for the control of reproduction

  (b) progestogens appear to exert many of their actions by preventing a rise in gonadotrophin secretion

  (c) progestogens have a negative feedback effect upon the release of prolactin, and can reduce, to some extent, circulating concentrations of testosterone and oestrogen by their actions upon gonadotrophin secretion
- ❏ high doses of progesterone and progestogens are centrally sedative in action
- ❏ progesterone and progestogens are commercially available in a variety of formulations including oral therapy that must be given daily, and oily suspensions and implants that provide a slow release over several weeks or months

Adverse effects of progestogens

General

- ❏ many transient effects may follow the administration of progestogens including:

  (a) increased appetite

  (b) weight gain

  (c) lethargy

  (d) mammary enlargement

(e) occasional lactation (following the withdrawal of the agent)

(f) hair and coat changes

(g) temperament changes

❑ these effects vary in their incidence between the different progestogens, although in general they are less frequent with the more recently developed ones

❑ the subcutaneous administration of some progestogens (especially the depot preparations) may produce hair discoloration and local alopecia at the site of injection

❑ it is therefore recommended that administration should be performed in an inconspicuous site, although this is usually impractical

❑ all progestogens may potentially induce the production of growth hormone. Chronic over-secretion of growth hormone may result in the clinical signs of acromegaly and peripheral insulin antagonism which may result in diabetes mellitus

❑ progestogen therapy may also produce adrenocortical suppression

Specific adverse effects in the bitch

❑ progestogens may result in the development of cystic endometrial hyperplasia and pyometra (see 14.5)

❑ the risk is related to the particular progestogen used, as well as the amount administered, and the duration of treatment

❑ this action appears to be potentiated by oestrogen, and for this reason certain depot progestogens (medroxyprogesterone acetate) are not licensed for use when oestrogen concentrations are elevated (they are therefore not used for the suppression of oestrus)

❑ other depot progestogens (proligestone and delmadinone acetate) have been shown to be safe when administered at practically any stage of the oestrous cycle

❑ there are no preparations recommended for use on the first oestrous period or in pre-pubertal bitches

❑ benign mammary nodules can be induced by progestogen therapy, and it has been suggested that progestogens may induce mammary neoplasia, although this does not appear to be the case with proligestone

❑ progestogen therapy during pregnancy may delay or prevent parturition, and may produce masculinized female and cryptorchid male fetuses (see Chapter 16)

Specific adverse effects in the dog

❑ high doses of progestogens cause marked changes in semen quality, the majority of which are related to a direct effect upon the epididymides

❑ changes in semen quality may result in infertility

❑ however, it is surprising that lower doses administered for short periods of time produce no measurable effect on semen quality or fertility

Clinical use of progestogens in bitches

Control of oestrus (see Chapter 23)

❑ administration of progestogens to bitches in anoestrus prevents gonado-trophin secretion increasing above basal values, and therefore prevents a return to cyclical activity
❑ if given when there is follicular activity (pro-oestrus or early oestrus), ovulation is inhibited and the bitch returns relatively quickly to anoestrus
❑ when progestogens are given daily or as a depot preparation they mimic a luteal phase, which is followed by a state of anoestrus
❑ progestogens are generally administered in one of four regimes to control oestrus in the bitch

Subcutaneous administration of depot preparations during anoestrus

❑ depot progestogens (medroxyprogesterone acetate, delmadinone acetate, and proligestone) administered subcutaneously during anoestrus will prevent a subsequent oestrus and regular repeated dosing (at 4–6 month intervals) can be used to prevent oestrus on a long term basis
❑ medroxyprogesterone acetate and proligestone are licensed for this purpose
❑ delmadinone acetate is unlicensed and has to be administered more frequently because of its shorter duration of action
❑ it may be inadvisable to prevent oestrus for more than 2 years
❑ when therapy is ceased most females cycle normally
❑ progestogens may induce cystic endometrial hyperplasia and therefore reduce fertility

Oral administration of progestogens during anoestrus

❑ low doses of orally active progestogens (megestrol acetate, medroxyprogesterone acetate, altrenogest, norethisterone acetate) can be used to prevent oestrus for as long as administration is continued
❑ megestrol acetate and medroxyprogesterone acetate are licensed for this purpose
❑ should the animal enter pro-oestrus during the first few days of treatment, the dosage can be increased
❑ a period of anoestrus usually follows therapy, so oestrus does not return immediately after cessation of treatment

Oral administration of progestogens during pro-oestrus

❑ high doses of orally active progestogens (megestrol acetate, medroxyprogesterone acetate, altrenogest, norethisterone acetate) may be given during pro-oestrus to suppress the signs of oestrus
❑ megestrol acetate and medroxyprogesterone acetate are licensed for this purpose

❏ usually the signs of pro-oestrus/oestrus disappear within approximately 5 days
❏ treatment during late pro-oestrus may not prevent ovulation in the bitch, although conception is unlikely to occur
❏ treatment too early may lead to a return to oestrus soon after dosing
❏ a reducing dose regime administered from the first signs of pro-oestrus and continued for up to 16 days is usually efficacious
❏ this is usually followed by a variable period of anoestrus; oestrus returns between 4 and 6 months after the end of medication

Subcutaneous administration of depot preparations during pro-oestrus

❏ administration of the new generation depot progestogens (proligestone) to bitches in early pro-oestrus may be used to suppress the signs of that oestrus
❏ older generation progestogens (medroxyprogesterone acetate) which have potent effects upon the uterus are not recommended
❏ signs of pro-oestrus/oestrus disappear within approximately 5 days
❏ following the depot progestogen, there is a variable anoestrus, and oestrus returns approximately 6 months later
NB: other agents that may be used for the control of oestrus cyclicity include long term administration of androgens commencing in anoestrus

Treatment of pseudopregnancy (see 2.7, 17.8)

❏ administration of progestogens to bitches with clinical signs of pseudo-pregnancy produces a suppression of prolactin secretion and the clinical signs rapidly disappear
❏ prolactin concentration is reduced for the duration of progestogen administration
❏ prolactin may increase again if progestogen therapy is rapidly withdrawn
❏ progestogens may be administered either orally daily (for example, megestrol acetate) or by depot injection (for example, proligestone or delmadinone acetate)
❏ first generation progestogens such as medroxyprogesterone acetate are not recommended because they have marked effects upon the uterus and might potentiate the development of a pyometra
❏ oral therapy is often associated with relapse of the clinical signs, if therapy is terminated too quickly; this can usually be prevented by gradually reducing the dose over a period of approximately 7 or 10 days
❏ care must be taken to ensure that the bitch is not pregnant, especially if depot progestogens are to be used because these can delay or prevent parturition
❏ it is likely that the return to oestrus will be delayed following the administration of progestogens
NB: other options for the treatment of pseudopregnancy include the administration of androgens, oestrogens, or combinations of these, or the use of prolactin antagonists such as bromocriptine or cabergoline

Treatment of mammary tumours

❑ both oestrogen and progesterone receptors have been identified in canine mammary tumours
❑ until recently some clinicians have used progestogen therapy (megestrol acetate) for the control of oestrogen-dependent mammary tumours
❑ therapy is empirical, and may not be efficacious because many advanced tumours possess few steroid receptors and appear to have an autonomous growth pattern
❑ care should be taken if progestogen use is contemplated because these agents may promote mammary neoplasia

NB: other agents that may be used to control mammary tumours include androgens, and the anti-oestrogens such as tamoxifen

Treatment of habitual abortion (see 19.5)

❑ there is only anecdotal evidence that habitual abortion occurs in the bitch
❑ it is therefore not appropriate to supplement bitches with progestogens to prevent habitual abortion
❑ progestogen supplementation during pregnancy may produce masculinized female pups, cryptorchid male pups, and may possibly impair or delay parturition resulting in fetal death

Clinical use of progestogens in dogs

Antisocial behaviour and other behavioural problems

❑ aggression, roaming, territory marking, copulatory activity, destruction and excitability exhibited by both entire and castrated dogs may be controlled in some cases by progestogens
❑ their actions relate both to their anti-androgenic effect and their central sedative action
❑ depot progestogen therapy may need to be repeated every month for the shorter acting preparations (delmadinone acetate) and up to every 6 months for the longer acting preparations (medroxyprogesterone acetate and proligestone)
❑ oral therapy has also been shown to be effective and has the advantage that the dose may be adjusted to the effect

NB: behaviour modification training is an essential adjunct to progestogen therapy, and entire dogs should be considered for castration

Benign prostatic hyperplasia (see 15.7)

❑ progestogens are both anti-androgenic and have a direct effect upon the prostate gland
❑ these actions are responsible for the rapid reduction in the clinical signs associated with regression of the prostate gland

❏ depot therapy usually causes remission of clinical signs within 4 days, although a second treatment may be necessary in some individuals
❏ delmadinone acetate is commonly used because of its short period of action and its relative sparing effects upon sperm production
❏ other depot or orally active progestogens are equally efficacious and high doses or long treatment periods are necessary to interfere with fertility
❏ in dogs not required for breeding, castration is the treatment of choice

NB: other agents that may be used for the treatment of benign prostatic hyperplasia include oestrogens and anti-androgens such as flutamide and finasteride

Prostatic neoplasia (see 15.7)

❏ some clinical improvement may be seen in dogs with prostatic neoplasia following the administration of progestogens
❏ the effect is usually only short-term, and progestogens offer little relief in metastatic disease

NB: other agents that may be used include oestrogens, anti-androgens such as flutamide and finasteride, and gonadotrophin releasing hormone (GnRH) analogues such as buserelin

Circum-anal adenomata

❏ the anti-androgenic effect of progestogens given as a depot or oral preparation is useful for causing temporary reduction in the size of these benign tumours
❏ tumours with central necrosis may not respond well
❏ in dogs not required for breeding, castration is the treatment of choice

NB: other agents that may be used include oestrogens

Contraception

❏ long term administration of high doses of progestogens may be useful to cause spermatozoal abnormalities and a possible suppression of spermatogenesis
❏ the concurrent administration of depot androgens appears to be more efficacious and allows the progestogen dose to be reduced
❏ castration is the method of choice in dogs that are not required for breeding

Epilepsy

❏ castration and/or progestogen therapy has been used for the control of some epileptiform convulsions
❏ the actions of progestogens may be related to their central sedative effect
❏ delmadinone acetate is licensed for this purpose, although other progestogens may be useful

24.2 OESTROGENS

- ❑ oestrogen is produced by ovarian follicles of the bitch, and the Leydig cells of the dog
- ❑ endogenous oestrogens are responsible for the development of the female sexual characteristics
- ❑ oestrogens are necessary for normal secretion and functioning of the uterine tubes, and changes in oestrogen concentration regulate the gonadotrophin surge which stimulates ovulation
- ❑ oestrogen is involved in the initiation of parturition
- ❑ in the male, oestrogens are involved in the feedback control of Leydig cell function
- ❑ high doses of exogenous oestrogen cause a negative feedback at the hypothalamic–pituitary axis and subsequent suppression of gonadotrophin secretion
- ❑ low doses of oestrogen enhance the release of FSH

Adverse effecs of oestrogens

General

- ❑ oestrogens have been shown to produce a dose-related bone marrow suppression
- ❑ this may result in a severe and possibly fatal anaemia and thrombocytopaenia
- ❑ prolonged oestrogen therapy may produce a non-pruritic bilaterally symmetrical alopecia and skin hyperpigmentation

Specific adverse effects in the bitch

- ❑ oestrogens potentiate the stimulatory effect of progesterone on the uterus, cause cervical relaxation and allow vaginal bacteria to enter the uterus
- ❑ oestrogen administration may therefore result in the development of cystic endometrial hyperplasia and pyometra (see 14.5)
- ❑ large doses of oestrogen may stimulate signs of oestrus in both entire and ovariohysterectomized bitches
- ❑ oestrogens may cause cervical relaxation and abortion in the pregnant bitch
- ❑ administration during pregnancy may cause congenital defects in the developing fetuses (see Chapter 16)

Specific adverse effects in the dog

- ❑ oestrogens may result in abnormalities of semen quality and a resultant reduction in fertility
- ❑ prolonged therapy may cause reversible prostatic metaplasia (see 15.7)

Clinical use of oestrogens in the bitch

Unwanted mating (see 23.7)

❏ oestrogens alter zygote transport time and impair implantation when administered soon after mating
❏ oestrogens may also produce a short luteal phase by interfering with luteinizing hormone (LH) support of the corpora lutea
❏ diethylstilboestrol, oestradiol cypionate and mestranol have been widely ued to treat unwanted matings
❏ only oestradiol benzoate is licensed for the treatment of unwanted mating in the UK
❏ oestradiol benzoate may be administered once at a relatively high dose within 4 days of mating, or at a lower dose 3 and 5 (and possibly also 7) days after mating
❏ the low dose regime has been advocated in an attempt to reduce the possibility of adverse effects; both regimes appear efficacious
NB: other treatment options are to induce resorption or abortion by the use of prostaglandins, prolactin antagonists or combinations of these after pregnancy has been diagnosed

Pseudopregnancy (see 2.7, 17.8)

❏ oestrogens may be used to produce an inhibition of prolactin secretion in bitches with pseudopregnancy
❏ a preparation of ethinyl oestradiol combined with methyltestosterone is available and produces a good clinical response, although the dose suggested seems arbitrary
❏ recurrence of the clinical signs may follow abrupt termination of treatment
NB: other treatment options include the administration of progestogens, androgens or specific prolactin antagonists such as bromocriptine and cabergoline

Juvenile vaginitis (see 14.3)

❏ the condition usually regresses after the first oestrus
❏ if the clinical signs are severe some control may be effected using low doses of oral oestrogens daily for 5 days
❏ an alternative therapy is the topical application of oestrogen-containing creams

Oestrus induction (see 21.4)

❏ low doses of oestrogen enable follicle stimulating hormone (FSH) to stimulate the formation of LH receptors on granulosa cells
❏ diethylstilboestrol may be used orally daily for up to 2 days after the onset of pro-oestrus

❑ ovulation is ensured by the administration of human chorionic gonadotrophin (hCG)

NB: other treatment regimes include the administration of equine chorionic
gonadotrophin (eCG) combined with human chorionic gonadotrophin, or the
use of prolactin antagonists such as bromocriptine and cabergoline

Urinary incontinence

❑ in ovariohysterectomized bitches incontinence may relate to changes in the
   thickness of the urethral mucosa in the absence of oestrogen
❑ some cases respond to oestrogen therapy, whilst in others the response is
   short lived or absent

NB: other agents that may be used include the drugs that act directly upon the
urethral muscle such as phenylpropanolamine

Clinical use of oestrogens in the dog

Antisocial behaviour and other behavioural problems

❑ oestrogens may be useful in dogs which show antisocial behaviour
❑ the potential adverse effects result in progestogens being more commonly
   used

Benign prostatic hyperplasia (see 15.7)

❑ repeated administration of oestrogens will result in a reduction in prostatic
   size and the amelioration of the clinical signs
❑ the treatment of choice is probably low dose progestogens which have a
   minimal effect on fertility, or castration in the animal that is not required for
   breeding
❑ prolonged oestrogen therapy may result in prostatic metaplasia and a
   resultant increase in the size of the prostate gland

NB: other treatment options include the use of anti-androgens and GnRH
agonists

Prostatic neoplasia (see 15.7)

❑ clinical signs of prostatic neoplasia may be controlled in the short term by the
   administration of oestrogens
❑ progestogens may also be useful in the short term, whilst in man anti-
   androgens and GnRH analogues are widely used

Circum-anal adenomata

❑ the anti-androgenic effect of oestrogens may be useful to cause a decrease in
   the size of these tumours

NB: other options are the administration of progestogens, although the treatment
of choice is castration in dogs that are not required for breeding

24.3 ANDROGENS

❏ the naturally occurring androgens testosterone and dihydrotestosterone, are produced by the interstitial cells of the testes
❏ in the male, androgens mediate the development and maintenance of primary and secondary sexual characteristics and normal sexual behaviour and potency
❏ androgens play an important role in the initiation and maintenance of spermatogenesis
❏ androgens are generally not present in significant concentrations in the non-pregnant female
❏ androgens have a negative feedback effect upon the hypothalamic–pituitary axis, and will influence, among other things, the release of the gonadotrophins and prolactin
❏ synthetic androgens have a duration of their activity related to the nature of the ester

Adverse effects of androgens

General

❏ androgen therapy may produce virilizing effects such as aggression, and their use may be contra-indicated in dogs with existing behavioural problems
❏ in pre-pubertal animals premature epiphyseal growth plate closure may occur
❏ androgens are contra-indicated in nephrotic conditions because the anabolic component causes both sodium and water retention

Specific adverse effects in the bitch

❏ prolonged androgen administration may result in clitoral hypertrophy, and very rarely the development of an os clitoris
❏ repeated or prolonged therapy may result in a persistent vaginitis
❏ severe urogenital abnormalities may develop in female fetuses if androgens are administered to bitches during pregnancy (see Chapter 16)

Specific adverse effects in the dog

❏ high doses of androgen produce severe changes in spermatozoal morphology and fertility

Clinical use of androgens in the bitch

Control of oestrus (see Chapter 23)

❏ androgens may be administered to bitches in anoestrus to prevent a return to cyclical activity

❑ androgens are not useful for inhibiting oestrus in females with follicular activity (pro-oestrus or early oestrus)
❑ administration must commence in late anoestrus, at least 30 days before the onset of pro-oestrus
❑ they do not mimic the luteal phase, and there is no subsequent anoestrus; therefore cyclical activity returns rapidly after the cessation of treatment
❑ in the UK the most common regime is the administration of depot androgens during anoestrus either as a prolonged release implant, or depot injection of mixed testosterone esters; it is not uncommon for depot therapy to be supplemented by daily oral therapy
❑ in other countries an orally active synthetic androgen, mibolerone, is available
NB: other agents that may be used to control oestrus include the progestogens

Pseudopregnancy (see 2.7, 17.8)

❑ relatively high doses of androgens may be used to produce an inhibition of prolactin secretion
❑ this results in a rapid resolution of the clinical signs
❑ androgens may be more useful than either progestogens or oestrogens because they do not have any adverse effects on the uterus
❑ oral methyltestosterone or parenteral testosterone esters are efficacious; however, an orally active licensed preparation of methyltestosterone combined with ethinyl oestradiol is available which produces a good clinical response
NB: other treatment options for pseudopregnancy include the administration of progestogens, oestrogens alone, or specific prolactin antagonists such as bromocriptine and cabergoline

Mammary tumours

❑ androgens may be useful for the control of certain mammary tumours
❑ the action is related either to a negative feedback upon gonadotrophin release or to a direct local anti-oestrogenic effect
❑ therapy is empirical, and may not be efficacious because many advanced tumours possess few steroid receptors and appear to have an autonomous growth pattern
NB: other agents that may be used to control mammary tumours include the anti-oestrogen such as tamoxifen

Clinical use of androgens in the dog

Poor libido (see 18.2)

❑ there is no evidence in the dog that poor libido is caused by low circulating androgen concentrations
❑ androgens should not be used in these cases because they produce significant changes in spermatozoal morphology and fertility

NB: other agents that may be useful in dogs with poor libido include hCG which produces an increase in endogenous testosterone concentration

Poor semen quality (see 15.3, 18.3)

❏ androgen supplementation is commonly used in these cases, and this may produce disastrous results because the androgens suppress spermatogenesis via the negative feedback mechanism
❏ an analogue of dihydrotestosterone, mesterolone, is available in the UK for human use and is unusual in that it is not aromatized to oestradiol and does not significantly suppress the release of pituitary gonadotrophins

NB: other agents that may be useful in dogs with poor semen quality include the anti-oestrogens

Contraception

❏ long term administration of high doses of androgens may be useful for reducing semen quality
❏ the concurrent administration of progestogens appears to be more efficacious

Cryptorchidism (see 15.3)

❏ medical therapy with androgens has not been shown to be efficacious and is unethical

24.4 GONADOTROPHINS

❏ the gonadotrophins FSH and LH are secreted by the anterior pituitary gland
❏ in the bitch, FSH stimulates initial follicular development and its surge release is associated with the process of ovulation
❏ in the bitch, LH also stimulates follicular growth, is the trigger for ovulation and is a principal luteotrophic agent
❏ in the dog FSH stimulates spermatogenesis indirectly by an action upon the Sertoli cells, and LH stimulates the Leydig cells to produce testosterone
❏ neither FSH or LH are available for use in the dog; however
   (a) equine chorionic gonadotrophin (eCG) is mainly FSH-like in activity
   (b) human chorionic gonadotrophin (hCG) is primarily LH-like in effect

Adverse effects of gonadotrophins

General

❏ there is a risk of inducing anaphylactoid reactions and antibody formation following the injection of these protein preparations

Specific adverse effects in the bitch

❑ eCG if given to oestrous bitches may cause luteinization of follicles and interfere with ovulation

❑ hyperstimulation of the ovary by the administration of high doses or the use of repeated therapy may result in non-ovulating follicles and persistent oestrus behaviour

❑ a persistent elevation in plasma oestrogen concentration may lead to adverse effects typical of oestrogen toxicity

Specific adverse effects in the dog

❑ none

Clinical use of gonadotrophins in the bitch

Induction of oestrus (see 17.5, 21.4)

❑ repeated doses of eCG given to anoestrous bitches stimulate follicular growth and the production of oestrogen

❑ ovulation may occur spontaneously, following an endogenous surge of LH, or may be induced using hCG

❑ care must be observed when using eCG and hCG combinations because endogenous hyperoestrogenism may occur and result in inhibition of implantation, bone marrow suppression and death

❑ low doses of gonadotrophins are suggested to produce more physiological plasma oestrogen profiles

❑ a relatively low plasma progesterone concentration or short luteal phase following gonadotrophin-induced oestrus is common

NB: other agents that may be useful for the induction of oestrus include low dose oestrogens, or prolactin antagonists such as bromocriptine and cabergoline

Delayed puberty (see 17.1)

❑ therapy to induce oestrus may be attempted using an eCG/hCG regime

Hastening of ovulation (see 17.4)

❑ bitches that repeatedly fail to conceive are sometimes given hCG at the time of mating on the assumption that ovulation has not occurred or that early development of the corpora lutea is inadequate; there is no evidence that this is the case, and such 'blind' therapy cannot be recommended

❑ some bitches may have prolonged pro-oestrus or oestrus and the administration of hCG may possibly hasten ovulation; hCG is administered when more than 90% of vaginal epithelial cells are anuclear, or when a slight rise in plasma progesterone concentration has been detected

❑ premature administration of hCG may result in follicular luteinization and failure of ovulation

NB: GnRH may be used in a similar manner to hasten ovulation

Identification of ovarian tissue (see 4.9)

❏ it may be difficult to determine clinically whether a bitch has been ovario-hysterectomized
❏ the administration of hCG to bitches with ovaries results in an increase in plasma oestrogen concentration
❏ this method may therefore be clinically useful for detecting the presence of ovaries

NB: the administration of GnRH may also be clinically useful for the identification of spayed bitches

Clinical use of gonadotrophins in the dog

Diagnosis of testicular tissue (see 9.14)

❏ in male dogs with no scrotal testes the presence of testicular tissue can be confirmed by performing an hCG stimulation test (see 9.14)
❏ plasma testosterone concentration is measured before and 60 minutes after the intravenous administration of hCG; a significant rise in testosterone concentration is diagnostic of testicular tissue

Cryptorchidism (see 15.3)

❏ testicular descent will not occur following the administration of gonado-trophins
❏ the condition is likely to be inherited and medical treatment is unethical

Hypogonadism (see 18.1)

❏ treatment with gonadotrophins is not successful

Poor libido (see 18.2)

❏ a transient increase in libido may follow the administration of hCG to male dogs
❏ this effect is the result of increased endogenous testosterone concentrations

24.5 GONADOTROPHIN RELEASING HORMONE (GnRH) AGONISTS AND ANTAGONISTS

❏ GnRH controls gonadotrophin synthesis via a neuroendocrine mechanism
❏ several synthetic GnRH agonists are available, although none are licensed for use in the dog:
  (a) these agents cause an increase in the production of FSH and LH
  (b) however, their repeated administration results in a down-regulation of the receptors thus preventing the release of FSH and LH
❏ GnRH antagonists produce a reduction in circulating gonadotrophins within a few hours

Adverse effects of GnRH agonists and antagonists

General

❑ no general adverse effects have been reported with these agents in dogs

Specific adverse effects in the bitch

❑ repeated administration of both GnRH agonists and antagonists may result in absence of oestrus

Specific adverse effects in the dog

❑ repeated administration of both GnRH agonists and antagonists may cause a reduction in libido, and long term administration may cause reduced spermatozoal morphology and fertility

Clinical use of GnRH agonists and antagonists in the bitch

Identification of ovarian tissue (see 4.9)

❑ the administration of GnRH to intact bitches produces an increase in LH and subsequent rise in plasma oestrogen concentration
❑ this test may be useful for the detection of bitches that have been ovariectomized or ovariohysterectomized because no rise in oestrogen occurs

NB: an alternative method is to administer hCG and monitor plasma oestrogen concentration, which increases in bitches with ovaries

Hastening of ovulation (see 17.4)

❑ single doses of GnRH may be useful to hasten ovulation in bitches that are in oestrus
❑ the use of hCG, however, may be more efficacious, although neither drug has been adequately evaluated for this purpose

Control of oestrus (see 23.6)

❑ analogues of GnRH, such as nafarelin, may be used to prevent reproductive cyclicity because they cause initial stimulation and then receptor down-regulation:
  (a) prevention of oestrus may be achieved using subcutaneously implanted sialastic devices providing a sustained release of GnRH for up to 1 year
  (b) suitable preparations of these agents are not commercially available
❑ GnRH antagonists may be used to prevent cyclical activity when administered during pro-oestrus

NB: other agents that may be used to control oestrus include progestogens and androgens

Unwanted mating (see 23.7)

❏ the down-regulation effects of continuous GnRH administration may be used in attempt to withdraw gonadotrophin support of the corpus luteum
❏ similarly the daily administration of GnRH antagonists successfully suppresses luteal function:
  (a) a single dose of detirelix produces resorption or abortion depending upon the stage of pregnancy
  (b) administration very early in the pregnancy is, however, not efficacious even when the drug dose is increased
NB: other agents that may be used to induce resorption or abortion include oestrogens, prostaglandins, prolactin antagonists and progesterone antagonists

Clinical use of GnRH agonists and antagonists in the dog

Contraception

❏ both GnRH agonists and antagonists may be useful for the suppression of LH and FSH, causing a reduced libido and infertility
❏ in particular, depot preparations appear to be useful as reversible methods of contraception
NB: other products such as progestogens, androgens or progestogen–androgen combinations are readily available; castration is the method of choice in the animal that is not required for breeding

Prostatic disease (see 15.7)

❏ repeated or depot administration of GnRH agonists may be useful in dogs which have benign prostatic hyperplasia and prostatic neoplasia

24.6 PROSTAGLANDINS

❏ the reproductive prostaglandins are synthesized in the endometrium, and are luteolytic and spasmogenic in nature
❏ prostaglandins are involved in the termination of the luteal phase and the initiation of parturition
❏ there are no naturally occurring or synthetic prostaglandin analogues licensed for use in the bitch
❏ the naturally occurring prostaglandin $F_{2\alpha}$, dinoprost and several synthetic prostaglandin analogues (especially cloprostenol and luprostiol) have, however, been widely described

Adverse effects of prostaglandins

General

❏ prostaglandin administration may be followed by restlessness, hypersalivation, vomiting, abdominal pain, pyrexia, tachycardia, ataxia and diarrhoea
❏ high doses may be lethal

❏ these effects develop quickly after administration and usually persist for up to 60 minutes

Specific adverse effects in the bitch

❏ prostaglandin administration to pregnant bitches may cause resorption or abortion
❏ cases of closed-cervix pyometra given prostaglandin may develop uterine rupture

Specific adverse effects in the dog

❏ prostaglandins are not used in male dogs

Clinical use of prostaglandins in the bitch

Termination of pregnancy (see 23.7)

❏ low doses of dinoprost or cloprostenol given daily, or twice daily, for several days can be used to produce luteal regression
❏ repeated low doses cause lysis of the corpora lutea and induce abortion, especially when given later than 23 days after ovulation
❏ earlier treatment may not be efficacious because developing corpora lutea are more resistant to the effects of prostaglandin
❏ recent studies have, however, shown that daily treatment commencing 5 days after the onset of metoestrus (dioestrus) using high doses of prostaglandin may be efficacious, although adverse effects are common
❏ a better therapeutic option is to use a combination of prostaglandin and a prolactin antagonist such as bromocriptine or cabergoline, although the latter agents may also be used alone

Treatment of pyometra (see 14.5)

❏ prostaglandins may be used to induce uterine emptying (the result of their spasmogenic activity) and to remove the stimulatory effects of progesterone (the result of their luteolytic action)
❏ dinoprost administered at low doses twice daily for 5 days, combined with appropriate antibiotic and fluid therapy, may be used as a successful treatment
❏ following treatment approximately 20% of bitches return to fertility
❏ the long term complications include recurrence of pyometra, anoestrus, failure to conceive and abortion
NB: other agents that may be used to treat cases of pyometra include progesterone receptor antagonists such as RU486 and RU46534

Post-partum metritis (see 20.12)

❏ post-partum metritis in the bitch may be treated by using prostaglandins to induce uterine evacuation

❏ antimicrobial preparations are mandatory; however, in these cases there is no underlying hormonal component (plasma progesterone concentration is low) and therefore a rapid resolution should be expected
❏ a regime similar to that used for the treatment of pyometra may be employed
NB: other treatment options include the administration of oxytocin or ergometrine

Induction of oestrus (see 21.4)

❏ prostaglandins may be used to induce luteolysis; however, the luteal phase is followed by a variable period of anoestrus
❏ shortening of the luteal phase does not therefore produce a rapid return to oestrus
NB: methods of oestrus induction include the use of gonadotrophins, oestrogens and prolactin antagonists

Clinical use of prostaglandins in the dog

❏ there are no therapeutic roles for reproductive prostaglandins in the dog

24.7 OXYTOCIN AND ERGOT PREPARATIONS

❏ oxytocin receptors develop on the myoepithelial cells of the mammary gland shortly before parturition
❏ uterine oxytocin receptors also increase in number close to parturition, and oxytocin release stimulates contraction of the oestrogen-primed uterus
❏ several formulations of oxytocin and posterior pituitary extract are available commercially, and can be used to stimulate the smooth muscle of the mammary and genital tract
❏ ergotamines are alkaloid extracts of a rye fungus which are ecbolic agents:
  (a) they produce a prolonged spasm of uterine muscle
  (b) relaxation occurs only after 1 or 2 hours when the uterus then contracts rhythmically in a similar manner to that produced by oxytocin

Adverse effects of oxytocin

General

❏ there is a low incidence of skin sloughing or abscess formation recorded by some manufacturers following the subcutaneous administration of oxytocin
❏ ergot alkaloids may produce emesis and slight stimulation of the central nervous system

Specific adverse effects in the bitch

❏ oxytocin administration to a bitch in late pregnancy may initiate premature parturition

Specific adverse effects in the dog

❏ oxytocin and ergot preparations have no clinical indications in the dog

Clinical use of oxytocin in the bitch

Uterine inertia (see 20.1)

❏ cases of primary uterine inertia or secondary uterine inertia (following correction of the dystocia) may respond to parenteral oxytocin administration
❏ oxytocin has a short half-life and therefore repeated administration (every 15–30 minutes) may be necessary to maintain a clinical effect
❏ the use of a continuous low dose intravenous infusion does not appear to have been investigated in bitches
❏ oxytocin is contra-indicated in obstructive dystocia because uterine rupture may result
❏ ergot preparations may also be used in cases of inertia; however, they produce prolonged uterine contractions and are less suitable

Placental retention or fetal retention (see 20.11)

❏ oxytocin is usually effective at producing uterine contraction and expulsion of the pup and/or placenta
❏ the response to oxytocin rapidly decreases after parturition, and in cases that are presented late, a hysterotomy may be necessary
❏ ergot preparations may be used in these cases but are less efficacious because of the prolonged contractions that they produce

Post-partum haemorrhage (see 20.13)

❏ persistent haemorrhage may be controlled by oxytocin administration
❏ ergometrine may be a more useful agent in these cases because of the initial prolonged uterine contractions
❏ excessive haemorrhage, although very rare, may necessitate a hysterotomy to identify and correct the cause

Post-partum metritis (see 20.12)

❏ uterine evacuation may be induced by oxytocin administration in cases of post-partum metritis
❏ appropriate antibiotic therapy is mandatory
NB: other treatment options include the administration of prostaglandins or ergometrine

Sub-involution of placental sites (see 20.14)

❏ most cases regress spontaneously after the bitch has returned to oestrus
❏ oxytocin has little effect once the clinical signs are established, but some

anecdotal reports suggest that treatment at the time of parturition may prevent the condition from developing

Agalactia

❑ lack of milk production is rare in the bitch; this has no treatment
❑ an absence of milk letdown is relatively common; it can be treated by the administration of oxytocin
❑ oxytocin does not increase milk production

Clinical use of oxytocin in the dog

❑ there are no clinical applications for oxytocin therapy in male dogs

24.8 PROLACTIN ANTAGONISTS

❑ prolactin is the primary luteotrophic factor of the pregnant and non-pregnant luteal phase
❑ corpora lutea initially appear to be autonomous; prolactin concentrations increase from day 20 onwards, and are then maintained for the duration of the luteal phase
❑ prolactin antagonists cause a rapid decrease in prolactin concentration and a subsequent decline in plasma progesterone concentration
❑ prolonged prolactin suppression results in a termination of the luteal phase, and the bitch enters anoestrus
❑ continual administration of prolactin antagonists during anoestrus causes a return to oestrus sooner than anticipated; the mechanism of this oestrus-induction action is unknown
❑ bromocriptine and cabergoline are ergot derivatives that inhibit prolactin release by direct stimulation of dopaminergic receptors of prolactin-releasing cells in the anterior pituitary gland
❑ cabergoline appears to be a more specific agent that has less side effects attributable to dopaminergic stimulation of the central nervous system
❑ neither bromocriptine nor cabergoline are licensed for use in the dog in the UK
❑ cabergoline is licensed for use in the dog in Europe and is available as a human preparation in the UK

Adverse effects of prolactin antagonists

General

❑ dopaminergic stimulation may result in nausea and vomiting
❑ lethargy and occasional constipation may also be noticed
❑ the adverse effects of bromocriptine can be reduced by using the minimal effective dose and mixing the drug with food. Specific anti-emetics such as metoclopramide may prevent vomiting, but whilst they are clinically useful, their administration does not make pharmacological sense because they also work via dopamine receptors

Specific adverse effects in the bitch

❏ administration of prolactin antagonists during pregnancy may cause abortion
❏ repeated administration will result in a shortening of anoestrus and a return to oestrus

Specific adverse effects in the dog

❏ there are no clinical applications of prolactin antagonists in male dogs

Clinical use of prolactin antagonists in the bitch

Pseudopregnancy (see 2.7, 17.8)

❏ suppression of prolactin causes a rapid resolution of the clinical signs of pseudopregnancy
❏ bromocriptine has been used for this purpose for some time; however, its effect of causing vomiting is a common reason for owner non-compliance and cessation of treatment
❏ vomiting can be reduced by starting with a very low dose and increasing this gradually over several days until a clinical effect occurs. Mixing the drug with food, or the prior administration of metoclopramide may also be useful as discussed above
❏ cabergoline is widely available in Europe and has a higher activity, longer duration of action, and better tolerance, and produces less vomiting than bromocriptine
NB: other agents that may be used for the treatment of pseudopregnancy include progestogens, androgens, oestrogens and androgen–oestrogen combinations

Termination of pregnancy (see 23.7)

❏ repeated administration of the prolactin antagonists produces a reduction in plasma progesterone concentration and resorption or abortion
❏ both agents are more effective when given later in pregnancy because the role of prolactin is more important at this time
❏ efficacy can be increased, and treatment may be given earlier, when prolactin antagonists and prostaglandins are given simultaneously (see 23.7)
NB: other agents that may be used to terminate pregnancy include prostaglandins or progesterone antagonists

Induction of oestrus (see 21.4)

❏ apparently normal and fertile oestrous periods may be induced in anoestrous bitches following continual administration of bromocriptine or cabergoline
❏ the time to the onset of oestrus seems to relate to the stage of anoestrus; bitches in late anoestrus respond more quickly than those in early anoestrus.

Treatment starting in the luteal phase may also be effective but the treatment period is longer
❏ the induced oestrus appears to be physiological, and whilst the mechanism of action is uncertain it may be the result of inhibition of remnant progesterone production by the corpora lutea
NB: other agents that may be used to induce oestrus include low dose oestrogens or gonadotrophin combinations

Clinical use of prolactin antagonists in the dog

❏ there are no therapeutic roles for prolactin antagonists in the dog

24.9 PROGESTERONE ANTAGONISTS

❏ specific progesterone receptor antagonists have antiprogestogenic effects
❏ the availability of these agents varies from one country to another:
   (a) mifepristone (RU486) appears to be most widely obtainable; it is available as an orally active product, but sale is limited in some countries because of potential human misuse
   (b) aglepristone (RU534) has recently been marketed for use in bitches in France, and is available as an injectable solution
❏ administration of these agents produces no initial change in plasma progesterone concentration; however, progesterone action is blocked

Adverse effects of progesterone antagonists

General

❏ adverse effects following the administration of these products have not been reported

Specific adverse effects in the bitch

❏ administration of progesterone antagonists to pregnant bitches will result in resorption, abortion or premature parturition, depending upon the time of administration

Specific adverse effects in the dog

❏ there are no therapeutic uses of progesterone antagonists in male dogs

Clinical use of progesterone antagonists in the bitch

Pregnancy termination (see 23.7)

❏ the administration of mifepristone to pregnant bitches at 28 days after ovulation produces fetal death and resorption within 5 days of treatment
❏ earlier administration requires a longer treatment period

❑ in later pregnancy, mifepristone administration results in abortion, or premature parturition
❑ aglepristone may be used to terminate pregnancy at any stage, even immediately after ovulation

Pyometra (see 14.5)

❑ aglepristone administration on days, 1, 3, 5, 8 and 16 after presentation appears to be successful for the treatment of pyometra in the majority of dogs
❑ the use so far has been limited; however, the regime produced no adverse effects, and emptying of uterine fluid occurred quickly producing resolution of the clinical signs
❑ some of the bitches returned to normal fertility after treatment

Clinical use of progesterone antagonists in the dog

❑ there are no clinical indications for the use of progesterone antagonists in male dogs

24.10 SYNTHETIC ANTI-OESTROGENS

❑ these include clomiphene citrate and tamoxifen
❑ clomiphene citrate and tamoxifen are both antagonists at the hypothalamic receptor level; they displace oestrogen from the receptor and lead to a decreased negative oestrogen feedback
❑ as a result gonadotrophin release is increased; in humans this may result in follicular growth and ovulation
❑ peripheral receptor antagonism also occurs and this may be useful in conditions which are stimulated by oestrogen
❑ anti-oestrogens also have an important action on the uterus; they may interfere with normal endometrial maturation, and therefore prevent implantation
❑ these agents also inhibit progesterone production from the corpora lutea and therefore interfere with the luteal phase
❑ in males the enhanced secretion of LH and FSH may stimulate spermatogenesis and Leydig cell function; however, clomiphene has significant intrinsic oestrogenic activity which may directly impair spermatogenesis whilst tamoxifen has no such oestrogenic activity and may be more suitable in the male

Adverse effects of synthetic anti-oestrogens

General

❑ the anti-oestrogens have been reported to produce gastrointestinal disturbances in man

Specific adverse effects in the bitch

❏ a high incidence of pathological changes of the bitch's reproductive tract is induced by tamoxifen including ovarian cysts and endometritis; this drug cannot therefore be recommended for use in animals that are required for future breeding

❏ tamoxifen may produce some oestrogenic adverse effects including vulval swelling and discharge and attractiveness to male dogs; these effects may be mediated by an oestrogenic metabolite of tamoxifen

Specific adverse effects in the dog

❏ no male-specific abnormalities have been reported

Clinical use of synthetic anti-oestrogens in the bitch

Termination of pregnancy (see 23.7)

❏ tamoxifen has been shown to terminate pregnancy when given at relatively high doses twice daily during pro-oestrus, oestrus, or early metoestrus (dioestrus)

❏ the high incidence of adverse effects makes this regime unusable

NB: other agents that may be used for the termination of pregnancy include oestrogens, prostaglandins, prolactin antagonists and combinations of these

Mammary neoplasia

❏ there is little evidence of clinical response of canine mammary tumours to therapy with anti-oestrogens

❏ anecdotally, tamoxifen may control progression of the tumour; however, the high incidence of oestrogenic adverse effects results in therapy being withdrawn in a large number of cases

Clinical use of synthetic anti-oestrogens in the dog

Poor semen quality (see 18.3)

❏ in man, both clomiphene and tamoxifen have been reported to improve semen quality in cases of oligozoospermia

❏ tamoxifen is more widely used because of the intrinsic oestrogenic property of clomiphene which may directly impair spermatogenesis

❏ neither agent has been investigated for use in the dog

NB: other products which may be used in these cases include synthetic androgens such as mesterolone

24.11 SYNTHETIC ANTI-ANDROGENS

❏ anti-androgens may have several mechanisms of action:
   (a) cyproterone acetate is a progestogen which is principally anti-androgenic

(b) flutamide inhibits androgen uptake and/or nuclear binding of androgen
(c) finasteride is a specific 5α reductase inhibitor which prevents the conversion of testosterone into dihydrotestosterone
(d) formestane is an aromatase inhibitor which inhibits the conversion of androgen to oestrogen in peripheral tissue

Adverse effects of synthetic anti-androgens

General

❏ adverse effects of these agents have not been reported in dogs, but in man include nausea, gastrointestinal upsets and gynaecomastia

Specific adverse effects in the bitch

❏ these agents have no clinical indication in the bitch

Specific adverse effects in the dog

❏ prolonged anti-androgen administration may result in a reduction in semen quality and poor fertility

Clinical use of synthetic anti-androgens in the bitch

❏ there are no clinical indications for the use of these products in the bitch

Clinical use of synthetic anti-androgens in the dog

Benign prostatic hyperplasia (see 15.7)

❏ dogs with prostatic hyperplasia may respond to the administration of anti-androgens by a reduction in prostatic size and disappearance of the clinical signs
❏ the concern with the use of these products is that there may also be a reduction in fertility
❏ flutamide has been shown to reduce prostatic size with no change in libido or sperm output
❏ finasteride has been shown to produce a dramatic decrease in prostatic size and a reduction in the secretion of prostatic fluid; however, total spermatozoal output did not change and fertility remained unaltered
❏ formestane has not been evaluated for use in dogs
NB: other preparations that may be used to treat benign prostatic hyperplasia include progestogens and oestrogens

Prostatic neoplasia (see 15.7)

❏ anti-androgens have not been reported for use in cases of prostatic neoplasia; however, both flutamide, finasteride and formestane have been shown to be useful for the control of clinical signs in man

25 Ovariohysterectomy

❑ ovariohysterectomy (neutering) means removal of the uterus and both ovaries; this is the standard practice in the UK
❑ in bitches not intended for breeding this operation should be considered seriously because, in most cases, any disadvantages are far outweighed by the advantages (see Chapter 23 and 25.6); it also helps to reduce the massive problem of unwanted pups

25.1 INDICATIONS

❑ prevents problems associated with oestrus, i.e. discharge, repeated urination and unwanted attention of male dogs whilst exercising the bitch
❑ reduces nuisance and road traffic accidents caused by the bitch roaming and male dogs being attracted to the house
❑ prevents unplanned pregnancies
❑ prevents pyometra (see 14.5)
❑ should prevent false pregnancy (see 2.7 and 25.6)
❑ reduces incidence of mammary neoplasia (bitches which are neutered before the first oestrus very rarely develop mammary neoplasms)

25.2 TIMING

❑ spaying bitches before puberty is surgically easiest and should reduce the likelihood of operative complications
❑ however, it is said to increase the incidence of obesity, incontinence and 'juvenile' vulva (see 14.1), although this is not proven
❑ most authorities therefore advise spaying after the first oestrus

Timing after first oestrus

❑ about 20 days after oestrus; however, the blood supply to the uterus and ovaries is good at this time and haemostasis may be a problem. This may be a good time to spay a bitch which is not wanted for breeding and has been mated inadvertently (see 23.7)
❑ about 3 months after oestrus; by this time the ovaries (corpora lutea) have become inactive and blood supply is minimal. However, do not operate if a bitch is in false pregnancy as signs may recur post-surgically (see 2.7). Do not operate within 2 months after hormonal treatment for false pregnancy (see 24.1, 24.2, 24.3, 24.8)

❏   after parturition; a bitch can be spayed as soon as the puppies are completely weaned (6–8 weeks) and lactation has finished
❏   cases of pyometra must be operated on when the patient's chances of survival are greatest (see 14.5)

25.3 OPERATIVE TECHNIQUE

(1)   prepare for mid-line laparotomy
(2)   make a mid-line incision from the umbilicus caudally to just over half way between the umbilicus and the pubic brim
(3)   locate the uterus (horn) in the caudal abdomen with a finger or spay-hook; it lies against the dorso-lateral abdominal wall
(4)   exteriorize the horn and its attached broad ligament and follow it to its cranial (ovarian) pole
(5)   locate the ovary (roughly pea sized) with the thumb and index finger
NB: it is difficult to see the ovary due to fat in the ovarian bursa and surrounding tissue. Also the ovary is intra-abdominal at this stage
(6)   exteriorize the ovary; this is a difficult task but is easier if the bitch has been given a muscle relaxant. Gently pulling the ovary towards or through the abdominal incision allows identification of the suspensory ligament which is a tight band in the cranial border of the mesovarium. Its resistance is overcome by:
(a) pulling the ovary gently and slowly until the ligament is sufficiently stretched, or
(b) pulling the ovary until the ligament ruptures, or
(c) rupturing the ligament by putting two small haemostats on its cranial (free) edge and twisting them in opposite directions, or
(d) putting two transfixing ligatures around the ligament and sectioning between them
(7)   the ovarian vessels run in the mesovarium, but usually cannot be seen due to fat. Before ligation, the mesovarium is separated from the mesometrium by blunt pressure with a finger-tip or haemostat in an avascular area
(8)   ligate the ovarian vessels with absorbable material by one of the following methods:
(a) a single ligature proximal to the ovary: reflex bleeding from the genital tract is prevented by placing a haemostat across the proper ligament of the ovary, i.e. between the ovary and the tip of the uterine horn
NB: continued pressure must be applied to the first throw (double) of the ligature knot to ensure that it is as tight as possible – it *must* compress the ovarian vessels through the fat and sufficient space must be left between the ovary and the ligature to allow for an adequate piece of tissue to be left distal to the ligature to prevent its subsequent slipping. Also *all* the ovary must be removed
(b) two clamps, e.g. haemostats, are placed across the mesovarium. A ligature is applied proximal to both; the tissue is divided between the

clamps by cutting or by rotating the clamps in opposite directions and pulling them apart to tear the tissue
(c) the three clamp technique: three clamps are applied to the mesovarium. A ligature (first throw) is laid loosely in between proximal and middle clamps. The proximal clamp is then removed and the ligature tied in the groove which the clamp left. The mesovarium is severed as in (b)

(9) release the stump of the mesovarium by removing all clamps – it can be held with Allis tissue forceps and allowed to retract slowly whilst checking for haemorrhage

(10) the broad ligament (mesometrium), i.e. between its cranial end and the body of the uterus, can be:
(a) cut with scissors or torn: during this process the very tough round ligament (which runs from the proper ligament of the ovary to the internal inguinal ring in a fold of the mesometrium) is also severed. This procedure allows some bleeding which usually causes no problems clinically
(b) ligated: this is necessary in removal of distended or inflamed uteri. One or two ligatures are used to compress the whole broad ligament

(11) treat the other ovary and broad ligament in the same way
NB: the right ovary is more cranial than the left and is therefore more difficult to remove

(12) the distal uterus is best severed at the cranial vagina, but sometimes the cervix and part of the uterus are left. The uterine vessels run parallel with the uterine body, on both sides; these can be ligated separately with transfixing ligatures

(13) ligate the uterus/cervix with a transfixing ligature
NB: the ligature should not enter the lumen. The uterus is severed proximal to the ligature and allowed to retract into the abdomen slowly using Allis forceps to check for haemorrhage

(14) before and during closure of the abdominal incision, check for blood in the abdomen. This may be coming from:
(a) the ovarian vessels; to exposure the right ovarian stump, locate the mesoduodenum and hold it to the left; to expose the left ovarian stump, locate the mesocolon and hold it to the right
(b) the uterine vessels
(c) the broad ligament
(d) vessels in the abdominal wound

(15) young bitches may also be spayed through the flank in a manner similar to cats

25.4 OVARIAN TRANSPLANT TECHNIQUE

❏ because of the possible problems of spayed bitches becoming overweight and lethargic, the following operation has been suggested in working bitches:
(1) remove ovaries
(2) dissect from bursa

(3) slice into pieces about 2 mm thick
(4) make an incision through the serosa of the stomach on its greater curvature
(5) bluntly dissect a pocket between the serosa and muscularis
(6) put a piece of ovary in the pocket and suture the serosa
(7) repeat until all the ovary is transplanted

Theory

❑ if the ovarian tissue 'takes' it will function normally
❑ when follicles grow the oestrogen will reach the liver immediately and be conjugated there
❑ this will not allow free oestrogen into the peripheral circulation in sufficient quantities to cause signs of oestrus, but will ensure small amounts of oestrogen in the circulation

Disadvantages

❑ a high incidence of neoplasia and stomach ulceration at the site of transplantation has been reported and the technique cannot be recommended
❑ lengthy operation, incision needs to be more cranial than for normal spay, and is easiest done by two people
❑ does not prevent subsequent urinary incontinence
❑ may get mild signs of pro-oestrus and attraction to male dogs

25.5 OVARIOHYSTERECTOMY FOR PYOMETRA

❑ The operation is similar to that in the healthy bitch except that fluid and antibiotic therapy should be considered and:
(1) the swollen uterus is seen as soon as the abdomen is opened
(2) exteriorize the uterus carefully; it is very friable
(3) ligate the mesovarium
(4) ligate the broad ligament
(5) ligate the uterine vessel separately
(6) it is best to remove the uterus at the cranial vagina: ensure there is no spillage of pus into the abdomen by:
(a) packing the area with swabs
(b) sectioning between two clamps and wiping the vaginal stump with a clean swab which is then discarded
(c) oversewing the uterine stump; this is very difficult as the tissues are friable and may cause trapping of bacteria and granuloma formation or stump pyometra
(7) antibiotics may be applied to the uterine stump

25.6 POSSIBLE OPERATIVE AND POST-OPERATIVE COMPLICATIONS

Anaesthesia

❏ this is routine for healthy bitches but toxaemic animals, e.g. pyometra, are more at risk
❏ fluid therapy is mandatory in cases of pyometra

Haemorrhage

❏ ovarian vessels: poor ligation technique
❏ broad ligament: unlikely to be serious
❏ uterine vessels: can be fatal; usually due to uterine artery recoiling caudally out of ligature, i.e. due to stretching vagina forwards
❏ clotting defect

Treatment

❏ usually best not to re-explore the abdomen as the bitch is now a poor anaesthetic risk and the free blood in the abdomen makes tracing its source difficult
❏ use plasma expanders and/or blood intravenously with antibiotics and warmth

Wound breakdown

❏ inappropriate suture material or faulty technique
❏ self trauma by bitch (may need Elizabethan collar)

Haemorrhagic discharge per vaginam within 7 days

❏ usually due to a transfixing ligature being placed through the vaginal lumen

Treatment

❏ re-operate and remove the vaginal stump if bleeding persists after antibiotic treatment

Post-renal abscess with a discharging sinus in the flank

❏ due to using non-absorbable ligature material which was contaminated with bacteria

Treatment

❏ ensure that the sinus originates from the site of the ovarian pedicle by surgical dissection or contrast radiography: these sinuses may take up to a year to form but can have other sources
❏ remove the abscess by blunt and blind dissection via a mid line laparotomy; this can be very difficult

Post-spay oestrus due to leaving part of an ovary *in situ*

❏ ensure that the bitch is really in oestrus, i.e. by taking a vaginal smear; some bitches with vaginitis are thought to be in oestrus (see 4.5)
❏ perform a laparotomy immediately post-oestrus when the ovarian remnant is still large due to the corpora lutea

NB: aplasia of part of the uterus may occur (see 14.5): the ovaries are usually present but may be difficult to locate during ovariohysterectomy

Post-spay false pregnancy

❏ usually due to inappropriate timing of ovariohysterectomy (see 2.7 and 24.1, 24.2, 24.3, 24.8)
❏ it is only caused by an ovarian remnant if oestrus precedes false pregnancy after spaying

Obesity

❏ this is the most common post-spay problem
❏ some breeds are likely to put on weight anyway after middle age, e.g. labradors
❏ it is easier to prevent a dog from gaining weight than it is to reduce its weight
❏ in order to prevent weight gain:
   (a) advise the owner of this likelihood as often as possible
   (b) advise regular weighing of the bitch after spaying
   (c) consider the early use of 'obesity diets' if reduction of energy intake and increased exercise do not prevent weight gain

Change of coat texture

❏ for example, Irish setters, samoyeds, etc. These changes are unavoidable

Urinary incontinence (see 17.10)

❏ inability to control urination; this may be caused by:
   (a) atrophy of the urethral muscles and epithelium which allows the uncontrolled escape of urine, especially when the bitch is in lateral recumbency (see 24.2)
   (b) acquired ectopic ureter due to the ureter being inadvertently included in the uterine ligature and forming a fistula into the vagina; the possibility of this occurring seems very unlikely and cases have been recorded where laparotomy with no involvement of the urogenital tract has apparently 'triggered-off' incontinence due to an ectopic ureter

Pyometra

❏ occasionally, if the uterine body is not removed a pyometra can develop, i.e. a 'stump pyometra'

❑ this is probably very rare if the ovaries have also been removed
❑ treatment is as for pyometra
NB: neutered dogs and bitches can only be shown under Kennel Club rules if they have a registered litter or if the owner has a veterinary certificate to say that the operation was necessary for medical reasons; some exceptions may be made on individual application to the Kennel Club

25.7 OVARIECTOMY

❑ in many European countries ovariectomy rather than ovariohysterectomy is performed
❑ the surgical technique is more simple and can be performed quickly
❑ the uterus rapidly atrophies after the ovaries are removed
❑ uterine disease is uncommon unless the bitch is given exogenous reproductive steroids, e.g. progestogens for the control of skin disease, or oestrogens for the control of vaginitis

26 Orchidectomy

- orchidectomy (orchiectomy, castration, neutering, gelding) means removal of the testes; the epididymides are also usually removed
- traditionally it has been considered rational to neuter bitches but unnecessary to neuter dogs
- neutered male dogs make better pets because they are less likely to roam or be restless; neither can they father puppies

26.1 INDICATIONS

- reduces the incidence of many sex-linked antisocial habits, e.g. copulatory behaviour, roaming, urine marking and aggression to other male dogs (see Chapter 24)
  NB: castration rarely modifies aggression towards people
- testicular tumours (see 15.3)
- testicular torsion (see 15.3)
- severe trauma to scrotum and/or testes (see 15.3)
- cryptorchid and ectopic testes (see 15.3)
- prostatic disease (see 15.7)
- peri-anal adenoma (see 24.1, 24.2)
- perineal rupture

16.2 TIMING

Elective castration

- this may be carried out from 5 months; early castration may increase the likelihood of obesity

Castration for antisocial behaviour

- this may be carried out at any time; it is most effective for the prevention of roaming
- older dogs are more likely to have 'learned' behavioural patterns, i.e. they are no longer testosterone dependent
- castration may be preceded by progestogen treatment to assess the likely efficacy of surgery (see Chapter 24)

Cryptorchid and ectopic testes

- these are more likely to become neoplastic than scrotal testes
- they should be removed before the dog is about 3 years old

NB: unilateral cryptorchids are fertile and potent; bilateral cryptorchids are sterile and potent (see 15.3)

Strangulated and neoplastic testes

❏ these are removed when diagnosed

Perineal rupture

❏ the dog is castrated at the time of rupture repair

Anal adenomata and prostatic disease

❏ castration may be preceded by progestogen or oestrogen treatment to confirm that the conditions are androgen dependent (see 24.1 and 24.2)

26.3 OPERATIVE TECHNIQUE

Possible sites

❏ prescrotal in mid line; this is the best
❏ prescrotal lateral to mid line (one incision)
❏ prescrotal lateral to mid line (two incisions, one for each testis)
❏ scrotal: this is to be avoided because of haemorrhage, scrotal oedema and post-operative self trauma
❏ scrotal ablation: this is sometimes performed in adult dogs of the larger breeds; it is also necessary when the scrotum is traumatized (see 27.14)
❏ a caudal approach has been described in conjunction with repair of perineal ruptures

Preparation

❏ do *not* traumatize the scrotum during clipping
❏ do *not* scrub the scrotum
❏ do *not* apply strong antiseptics, e.g. povidone–iodine or methylated spirit to the scrotum; use sterile saline and dilute chlorhexidine
❏ *do* cover the scrotum with a drape

Procedure 1 (open castration)

(1) push one testis into a prescrotal position
(2) make a longitudinal incision through the skin over the testicle and about the same length as the testicle; incise the skin, dartos, fascia and parietal peritoneum (*tunica vaginalis communis*)
(3) expose the testis, epididymis and cord which are covered by and attached to the visceral peritoneum (*tunica vaginalis propria*)
(4) rupture by blunt dissection (finger pressure) the mesorchium (tunica vaginalis propria) close to where it is reflected as the tunica vaginalis communis, i.e. ensure that the blood vessels (spermatic artery and pampi-

niform plexus of spermatic veins) and ductus deferens (with the deferential vessels) are isolated in a common bundle (the spermatic cord)

(5) ligate the spermatic cord and sever:
(a) use absorbable ligatures
(b) ensure that the ligature is very tight; the ligature can be transfixed, but there is very little connective tissue, and passing the needle through a blood vessel can cause a haematoma
(c) the ligature can be laid after first crushing the cord with a haemostat
(d) return the cord slowly into the abdomen with thumb forceps, checking for haemorrhage
(6) the testicle and epididymis are attached to the tunica vaginalis communis by the straight ligament of the epididymis
(a) this can be cut, but small vessels often ooze blood
(b) it is better to place a ligature round the whole of the tunica
(7) repeat for the other testis
(8) repair the skin wound

NB: subcuticular sutures reduce skin haemorrhage and cannot be removed by the dog

Procedure 2 (closed castration)

(1) incise skin, dartos and fascia: do *not* incise the parietal peritoneum
(2) bluntly dissect (with a dry swab) the fascia between the dartos and the tunica until the tunica (containing the testis and epididymis, etc.) is completely free of the scrotum
(3) ligate the cord (including the tunica vaginalis propria) with a double ligature or transfixing ligature

Advantage of procedure 2

❑ no direct opening is made into the peritoneal cavity thus preventing entry of infection and subsequent inguinal hernia (rare in the dog)

Disadvantage of procedure 2

❑ blunt dissection of the fascia can cause irritation
❑ it is possible for the spermatic vessels to slip out of the tunica after ligation
❑ the operation usually takes longer

26.4 POSSIBLE OPERATIVE AND POST-OPERATIVE COMPLICATIONS

Anaesthesia

❑ this is routine for healthy dogs; for older dogs the risk becomes greater

Haemorrhage

❑ from spermatic vessels: haemorrhage occurs into the abdomen and should

be treated as in the bitch (see 25.6); at laparotomy the ductus deferens is found dorsal to the bladder and ventral to the colon
❑ from the tunica vaginalis or subcutaneous tissues: this causes scrotal swelling (see below)

Scrotal swelling

❑ this is a common sequel because of the 'dead' space
❑ it is usually caused by blood and/or inflammatory fluid
❑ its occurrence can be minimized by strict haemostasis
❑ some practices ablate the scrotum of adult dogs of large breeds

Treatment

❑ antibiotics to prevent infection
❑ Elizabethan collar to prevent trauma to incision and scrotum
❑ assure the owner that the swelling is not due to growth of new testicles!

Wound breakdown

❑ due to faulty suture technique or self trauma by the dog
NB: castration wounds are very likely to be licked by the dog; some practices issue collars routinely

Aggression

❑ some owners worry that the dog may become more aggressive: this is not true
❑ the temperament change that occurs in most pets is desirable and not detrimental
❑ in working dogs, however, castration may significantly affect performance

Obesity

❑ not such a problem as in the bitch
❑ dogs that are castrated before puberty may develop a female-like shape

27 Other Common Surgical Procedures

27.1 CEASAREAN OPERATION (HYSTEROTOMY)

Indications (see Chapter 20)

- ❏ primary uterine inertia
- ❏ secondary uterine inertia
- ❏ unrelieved obstructive dystocia
- ❏ may be elective in achondroplastic breeds or where stenosis of the birth canal is known to exist
- ❏ elective where a fetal anomaly, e.g. anasarca, has been diagnosed by ultrasonography

Anaesthesia

- ❏ may consider administering intravenous fluids
- ❏ premedication is better avoided unless pups are known to be dead
- ❏ induction may be with:
  (a) methohexitone or propofol; these are rapidly metabolized by the dam
  (b) thiopentone; pups should not be removed for 15 minutes to allow metabolism by the dam
  (c) in small tractible dogs, isoflurane or halothane, nitrous oxide and oxygen may be delivered by face mask
- ❏ maintenance should be with isoflurane or halothane and oxygen

Surgical approach

Reasons why flank is not recommended

- ❏ more tissue damage is caused by incising muscles
- ❏ access to the uterus is limited
- ❏ the bitch may lie on wound when suckling

Reasons why mid line is the best approach

- ❏ good access to the uterus (a long incision can be made)
- ❏ the bitch can lie comfortably on both sides
- ❏ the pups do not interfere with the wound if the skin is closed with subcuticular sutures

Surgical technique

(1) exteriorize the whole uterus carefully: rough handling causes haematomata in the broad ligament

(2) for small litters make one incision in the uterine body; for large litters make an incision in the middle of each horn

(3) incise between adjacent placentae

(4) do not waste time trying to stop uterine bleeding; this will diminish as involution occurs

(5) force a pup to the incision and cut the amnion; the wet coat of the pup will prevent its skin from being damaged

(6) remove the pup, place a haemostat onto the umbilical cord close to the abdomen, sever the cord and hand the pup to an assistant

(7) ensure that traction on the cord does not cause an umbilical hernia

(8) gentle traction on the severed cord should cause separation of the allantochorion; if fresh blood is seen, e.g. when elective caesarean has been carried out too early, leave the fetal membranes

(9) if a dead pup, or one which is intravaginally positioned, is to be removed, try to reduce abdominal contamination by packing round the uterus with moist swabs

(10) close the uterine incision(s) with a Lembert or Cushing suture to invert the myometrium and appose the serosa

(11) wipe the uterus clean

(12) close the abdominal wound conventionally; subcuticular absorbable sutures in the skin protect the wound from attention by the pups

(13) oxytocin (1–2 IU/kg) (see 24.7) administration hastens uterine involution and evacuation of fluids

27.2 EPISIOTOMY

Indications (increase access to vagina)

❏ removal of vaginal tumours
❏ severing vaginal constrictions at the vestibulo-vaginal junction (see 14.3 and 27.4)
❏ removal of a prolapsed (hyperplastic) vagina (see 14.3 and 27.4)
❏ removal of large pup if vulva is small

Anaesthesia

❏ routine

Surgical approach

❏ perineal with the bitch in sternal recumbency and with the tail tied forwards

Surgical technique

(1) use diathermy
(2) incise the skin vertically from the dorsal commissure of vulva; identify and ligate larger bleeding vessels
(3) incise the caudal wall of vestibule deep to the skin incision
(4) afterwards close the vaginal wall with absorbable sutures so that knots lie between the vaginal wall and the skin
(5) close the perineal skin with simple interrupted sutures or inverted sutures of absorbable material

27.3 REMOVAL OF VAGINAL TUMOURS

Surgical approach

❑ may require episiotomy (see 27.2)

Surgical technique

(1) fibromata (polyps) are easily removed by ligating the pedicle; most originate in the vestibule
(2) benign submucosal tumours are usually easy to 'shell-out' after incising the mucosa
(3) locally malignant tumours involve the mucosa and successful removal is unlikely

27.4 SEVERING VESTIBULO-VAGINAL CONSTRICTIONS

Surgical approach

❑ usually requires episiotomy (see 27.2)

Surgical technique

(1) sever tissues as appropriate: haemostasis may be difficult
(2) some constrictions continue too far cranially to be completely broken down
(3) their extent may be predetermined by contrast vaginoscopy

27.5 REMOVAL OF PROLAPSED VAGINA BY SUBMUCOSAL RESECTION (see 14.3)

Surgical approach

❑ usually requires episiotomy (see 27.2)

Surgical technique

(1) catheterize the bladder and fix the catheter to a drape with forceps

(2)   identify the amount of vaginal floor (cranial to the urethral opening) to be removed, i.e. the base of the 'neck' of the prolapse

(3)   use diathermy

(4)   initially make a horizontal incision at the base of the prolapse, cranial to the urethral opening

(5)   only sever the mucosa: the junction between this and the submucosa is easily identified by its gelatinous (oedematous) appearance

(6)   continue the incision laterally on both sides and unite them dorsally

(7)   only identify and ligate/cauterize large vessels; capillary ooze may look severe but cannot be stopped and will diminish throughout surgery

(8)   due to the rugate nature of the vaginal floor, the incision will look uneven

(9)   peel the isolated patch of mucosa from the submucosa using a mixture of blunt dissection and diathermy

(10)   close the mucosal incision laterally with simple interrupted sutures of absorbable material with hidden knots

(11)   haemorrhage will diminish as closure proceeds

(12)   repair the episiotomy and remove the catheter

27.6 CORRECTION OF SEVERE VULVAL AND PERIVULVAL DERMATITIS

Indications

❑   persistent inflammation of the vulval labia and perivulval skin, particularly in the sulci or folds (see 14.1)

Surgical approach

❑   prepare the perineum and entire perivulval area

Surgical technique

(1)   identify the extent of the skin lesions; centrally this may extend to the vulval muco-cutaneous junction, peripherally it will be outside the peri-vulval skin fold

(2)   use diathermy

(3)   centrally, incise into healthy tissue inside the lesion: this may require removal of all the vulval labia and sometimes the clitoris

(4)   only ligate large vessels

(5)   laterally, incise into healthy skin all round the lesion

(6)   remove the diseased skin by blunt dissection and diathermy

(7)   appose healthy skin to vulva/mucosa laterally on both sides with a single suture

(8)   assess the likelihood that the skin can be apposed easily both dorsal and ventral to the vulva

(9)   excess skin at the wound margin may need to be removed to ensure that closure of the wound leaves no perivulval skin folds
        NB: it is unlikely that too much skin will be removed if the bitch is in

sternal recumbency; what appears to be stretching of skin in this position may still result in some skin folding when the bitch stands normally
   Ideally, post-surgically, there should be no skin folds (or sulci) round the vulva
(10) closure of wounds with subcuticular knots reduces wound breakdown due to the bitch licking at the site

27.7 CORRECTION OF CONGENITAL VULVAL ATRESIA (STENOSIS)

Surgical technique

(1) incise along medium raphe which connects the vulval labia
(2) suture the skin to the mucosa along the margins as necessary

27.8 REMOVAL OF OVARIAN TISSUE LEFT AFTER INCOMPLETE OVARIOHYSTERECTOMY

Indictions

❑ only operate if it can be confirmed that the bitch has truly been in oestrus by:
   (a) vaginal cytology during oestrus (see 4.5); erythrocytes may not be seen if the whole uterus has been removed
   (b) determination of plasma progesterone concentration 2 weeks after oestrus; elevated values indicate that ovulation has occurred (see 3.5)

Surgical technique

(1) mid-line laparotomy through the umbilicus, more cranial than for routine ovariohysterectomy
(2) locate the pad of fat in the remnant of the mesovarium, caudal to each kidney
(3) palpate the fat carefully on both sides; the presence of any hard structure indicates excision
(4) remove the intact fat pad as for routine ovariohysterectomy
(5) open the fat after removal, to confirm the presence of ovarian tissue
   NB: check both sides
(6) close the abdomen routinely

27.9 LOCATION AND REMOVAL OF ECTOPIC TESTES

Indications

❑ ectopic testes are those which do not occupy the normal scrotal position; in cryptorchids one or both testes are in the abdomen or inguinal canal (see 15.3)
❑ ectopic testes, particularly those that are intra-abdominal, are likely to become neoplastic

❏ because abnormal testicular descent is an inherited condition, it is often advised that any normally descended testis is also removed (see 26.1)

Surgical approach

Ectopic testes

❏ some ectopic testes may be palpated subcutaneously near the external inguinal ring
❏ a small skin incision reveals the testis which is usually embedded in a pad of fat
❏ removal is by simple ligation of the spermatic cord

Laparotomy

❏ this is performed by para-penile approach
❏ the transverse skin incision is started in the mid line, 1–2 cm cranial to the prepuce; 1–3 cm lateral to the penis it is extended caudally to the pubis
❏ subcutaneously, the pudendal vein and artery are identified, ligated and severed
❏ the penis is deflected laterally and a mid-line incision is made through the linea alba
❏ the bladder is located, exteriorized and reflected caudally
❏ this usually aids location of the vasa deferentia, which are white, hard tubular structures about 2 mm wide; they insert into the urethra after travelling a short distance through the prostate gland
❏ traction on the vasa deferentia usually results in exteriorization of the testes, although these may be visible immediately after incising the linea alba
❏ the mesorchium, which in this situation resembles the mesovarium but contains no fat, is ligated and sectioned, as is the vas deferens (including the deferential vessels)

Failure to find testes in the abdomen

❏ if no testis is located at the ab-urethral end of the vas deferens, this could be due to aplasia (only recorded once), the dog already having been castrated, or the testes having passed into or through the inguinal canal; in the last case:
(a) carefully remove the surgical drape on the side of the missing testicle
(b) gently pull rhythmically on the vas deferens
(c) the site of the testicle will be revealed by cutaneous movement above it
(d) the testis is likely to be under abdominal skin, in the femoral canal or lateral to the penis in the perineum
(e) even at this stage, it may be difficult for an assistant to identify the testis definitely by palpation
(f) surgically prepare and drape the site over the suspected position of the testis

(g) incise the skin and explore the subcuticular area; the testis is usually surrounded by fat

(h) ligate the spermatic cord, remove the tetis and close the skin incision

27.10 REMOVAL OF THE INTRA-ABDOMINAL GONADS IN INTERSEXUAL DOGS (see 16.6)

Surgical approach

❏   as for cryptorchid dogs (see 27.9) except that the skin incision may be mid line if there is no phallus in this area

Surgical technique

(1)   the tubular genital tract is identified by reflecting the bladder caudally
(2)   the gonadal attachment (mesorchium/mesovarium) to the abdominal wall is ligated and severed (it is usually fat-free)
(3)   any analogue of broad ligament is relatively non-vascular and can be torn
(4)   the tubular tract (uterus and/or vasa deferentia) is ligated close to its insertion into the urethra or vagina and removed
(5)   histological section of the gonads and tubular tract may reveal a variety of tissues

27.11 ENLARGING THE PREPUTIAL OPENING

Indications (see 15.1)

❏   phimosis: inability to expose the penis from the sheath
❏   paraphimosis: inability to retract the penis; this is sometimes not related to the size of the preputial orifice, and surgical enlargement is still followed by episodes where the exposed penis becomes engorged – the reason for this is unknown

Surgical technique

(1)   a longitudinal incision is made caudally from the preputial opening on the ventral aspect of the sheath
(2)   both skin and mucosa are incised; the extent of the incision should be judged by reference to a normal dog of a similar size; over-enlarging the orifice causes the penis to become dried and traumatized
(3)   the skin and mucosa are apposed with simple interrupted sutures

27.12 CORRECTION OF PERSISTENT PENILE FRENULUM (see 15.2)

❏   under general anaethesia the vental attachment (band of tissue) between the penis and sheath is severed with scissors; haemostasis is effected by direct pressure if necessary

27.13 AMPUTATION OF THE PENIS

Indications (see 15.1 and 15.2)

- ❏ non-healing wounds and ulcers
- ❏ tumours
- ❏ persistent penile exposure
- ❏ necrosis after congestion due to paraphimosis
- ❏ urination on chest and front legs
- ❏ constriction of the urethra due to callus formation after fracture of the os penis
- ❏ ulcerated/prolapsed urethra

NB: for persistent penile exposure and in dogs which urinate on their ventral abdomen and legs, operations to pull the prepuce forward have been described; in the author's experience they are not effective

Preparation

- ❏ dog in dorsal recumbancy
- ❏ prepare prescrotal area as for orchidectomy
- ❏ catheterize the bladder; this is essential but may be difficult if the urethra is occluded – use a narrow (6FG) catheter and stretch and gently rotate the penis from side to side
- ❏ occlude the distal end of the catheter
- ❏ retract the prepuce
- ❏ tie a 1 inch bandage tightly round the base of the penis, proximal to the bulbus glandis, with a reef knot
- ❏ tie the other end of the bandage to the table to restrain the penis in an upright position
- ❏ cleanse the glans penis gently with sterile saline and dilute chlorhexidine solution; do not use alcohol

Surgical technique

(1) identify the site of amputation, which must be proximal to the lesion; if possible it should be in the pars longa glandis

(2) amputations at or proximal to the bulbus glandis are very difficult due to the problem of dissecting the urethra from the urethral groove, which is deep at this location

(3) make a V-shaped incision on the ventral surface of the penis so that the point of the V is towards the dog

(4) make a similar incision on the dorsal surface so that the 'arms' of the Vs join laterally

(5) laterally and dorsally, incise through the corpus cavernosum to the os penis

(6) ventrally, carefully dissect the urethra from the urethral groove for about 2 cm distal to the incision; care must be taken not to damage the urethra by keeping the cutting edge of the blade towards the os penis

(7)   when the urethra is free from the groove of the os penis, make a circular incision around it (taking care not to cut through the catheter) about 2 cm distal to original incision

(8)   cut the os penis as proximally as possible using bone cutters

(9)   appose the integument laterally both ventral and dorsal to the urethra using continuous sutures of an absorbable material, e.g. 3/0 polyglycolic acid

(10) make a lateral longitudinal incision up the length of the exposed urethra

(11) fold the urethra back over the stump of the penis so as to cover it like an umbrella; the urethra will stretch to allow most of the stump to be covered

(12) anchor the urethra to the stump in several places with simple interrupted sutures, then complete its attachment with a continuous pattern

(13) remove the tourniquet (bandage); this may need to be cut carefully with scissors

(14) insert simple sutures over any bleeding points

(15) remove the catheter

(16) castrate the dog

Post-operative care

❏ bleeding, especially during urination, may be expected for some days
❏ an Elizabethan collar is advisable to prevent self trauma
❏ broad spectrum antibiosis should be administered
❏ subsequent stricture of the urethra is rare

NB: where lesions are close to the base of the bulbus glandis it is impossible to operate in this elective manner, although healing will sometimes occur satisfactorily despite inadequate urethral dissection and wound closure

27.14   SCROTAL ABLATION (WITH CASTRATION)

Indications

❏ sometimes carried out routinely when old or large dogs are castrated
❏ non-healing traumatic scrotal and/or testicular lesions
❏ pendulous scrotum due to testicular neoplasms

NB: scrotal ablation removes the dead space in which post-surgical blood and inflammatory fluid can accumulate

Preparation

❏ dog in dorsal recumbency
❏ complete hair removal from the scrotum and periscrotal area
❏ routine antiseptic cleansing of area

Surgical technique

(1)   tense the scrotum upwards, away from the dog

(2)   incise from the mid-line cranial to the scrotum to the mid-line caudal to the

scrotum with the middle of the incision curving away from the dog; this ensures adequate skin to close the wound but any excess can be removed later

(3)   repeat on the other side
(4)   incisions are deepened through the dartos, fascia and parietal peritoneum
(5)   individual bleeding vessels are ligated or coagulated with diathermy
(6)   the spermatic cords are ligated as in orchidectomy (see 26.3)
(7)   the scrotal septum is dissected by traction and incision
(8)   several subcuticular simple interrupted sutures with absorbable material, e.g. 2/0 polyglycolic acid, appose the skin
(9)   continuous subcuticular polyglycolic acid suture, or simple interrupted non-absorbable sutures (which require removal) can be used to close the skin

27.15 TESTICULAR BIOPSY

Indications

❏   confirmation of spermatogenic aberrations in dogs with poor semen quality
NB: testicular biopsy is not therapeutic and does not indicate a line of treatment; it is very useful in experimental investigation of male infertility

Preparation

❏   general anaesthetic
❏   cleanse the scrotum as for orchidectomy (see 26.3); do not use strong anti-septics or alcohol

Surgical technique

Needle biopsy

(1)   an assistant tenses the scrotum over the testis
(2)   make a 0.5 cm incision through the skin and dartos
(3)   insert the biopsy needle into the parenchyma of the testis
(4)   expose the inner cutting blades, rotate these and push the outer cannula over them
(5)   withdraw the needle and place the biopsy material into fixative, e.g. buffered formal saline or Bouin's fluid
(6)   the assistant applies constant pressure to the biopsy site with a surgical swab for 5 minutes
(7)   observe the scrotum closely after pressure is released; if swelling occurs (haematoma formation) pressure must be reapplied
(8)   the advantage of this technique is that it is relatively atraumatic; however, only a small piece of tissue is obtained. Sometimes there is no tissue in the needle and the procedure is repeated
(9)   if necessary, biopsies can be taken from several sites and both testes

Slice biopsy

(1)   easiest if an assistant holds the testicle tense in the prescrotal area, as for routine castration (see 26.3)
(2)   make a longitudinal incision about 1 cm long through the skin and parietal peritoneum
(3)   remove any fat that is obscuring the view of the testis
(4)   incise into the visceral peritoneal covering of the testis; this causes a bulge of parenchyma to protrude from the surface of the testis
(5)   remove the 'proud' tissue with a sharp scalpel or 'razor' blade and place in fixative
(6)   the testis can be moved and a second biopsy taken; the visceral peritoneum is closed with a continuous suture of fine absorbable material
(7)   the parietal peritoneum and skin are closed conventionally
(8)   the advantage of this technique is that larger pieces of tissue are obtained, but they are superficial and may not be representative of the testis; also damage is greater, and post-operative haemorrhage and trauma by the dog are more likely

27.16 URETHROTOMY

Indications

❏   removal of urethral calculi
❏   urethral stenosis due to stricture at the site of os penis fracture

Preparation

❏   dorsal recumbency
❏   prepare the area between the base of the os penis and the scrotum
❏   pass a urethral catheter if possible; if calculi are present they are usually at the base of the os penis and can be felt grating against the end of the catheter

Surgical technique

(1)   make a longitudinal incision over the site of the calculus or proximal to a stricture
(2)   the incision is continued until the calculus is felt under the blade, or urine escapes
(3)   remove all calculi if possible (their number and position may have been ascertained by radiography)
(4)   leave the urethrotomy open to heal by granulation; the dog will urinate both through the urethrotomy and distal urethra for a while
(5)   if the penile obstruction cannot be removed, the urethrotomy is converted to a urethrostomy by extending the skin and urethral incisions, and suturing urethral mucosa to skin on both sides with a continuous suture of, e.g. 2/0 polyglycolic acid

27.17 PROSTATIC BIOPSY

Indications

❏ usually to differentiate between prostatic neoplasia and other causes of prostatic enlargement/disease (see 15.7)

Surgical approach

Via laparotomy

❏ a wedge is removed from the enlarged and intra-abdominal prostate gland and the sides of the wound are closed with absorbable material

Para-rectal approach

(1) clip and prepare an area beside the anus
(2) incise the skin lateral to the anus with a pointed (no. 11) scalpel blade
(3) tense/hold the gland with one hand transabdominally and push a biopsy needle cranially from the para-anal incision with the other
(4) guide the needle into the gland and then rotate the blades to obtain a piece of tissue
(5) the advantage of the method is that it does not require a laparotomy; however, the procedure is blind and may rupture an abscess

Index

abortion, 142–6
  bacterial causes, 142–3
  habitual, progestagens and, 145, 188
  induction, 181–3, 191, 200, 204–5
    complications, 183
  partial, 145
  prevention of, 145–6
  of unknown aetiology, 145
  viral causes, 143
abscess
  post-renal, 213
  prostatic, 123
acrosome abnormalities, 56, 118, 161
activins, 44
adenomata
  ovarian, 108
  peri-anal, and orchidectomy, 189, 192, 216
afterbirth *see* placenta
agalactia, 203
aggression
  as indication for orchidectomy, 216
  following orchidectomy, 219
  reducing, using progestagens, 188
aglepristone, 107, 182, 205–6
alkaline phosphatase, 121
allantochorion, 77–8
allantois, 77
alopecia
  and progestagen, 185
  bilateral non-pruritic, 120
anabolic steroids, 61
anaemia
  and oestrogens, 190
  in pregnancy, 79
anal adenoma, 189, 192
anasarca, 150, 220
androgens, 15, 43, 193–5

  and prostatic disease, 122
  cause of enlargement of clitoris, 193
  contraception, 195
  control of oestrus, 193–4
  treatment of mammary tumours, 194
  treatment of poor libido, 194
  treatment of poor semen quality, 195
  treatment of pseudopregnancy, 194
androstenedione during metoestrus, 15
anoestrus, 10–11
  clitoral examination, 25
  endoscopic examination, 25
  ovaries in, 6
  primary, 131
  prolonged, 132
  uterus in, 5
  vagina in, 18
  vaginal cytology, 18
anorchia, 114
anorchism, 114
anorexia in pseudopregnancy, 133
anovulation, 132
anthelmintics, 90
anti-androgens, 207–8
  effects, 207
  side-effects, 208
  treatment of prostatic disease, 208
antibiotics
  in perivulval dermatitis, 96
  in prostatic disease, 123
  in pyometra, 106
anti-oestrogens, 206–7
  effects
  side-effects
  termination of pregnancy, 207

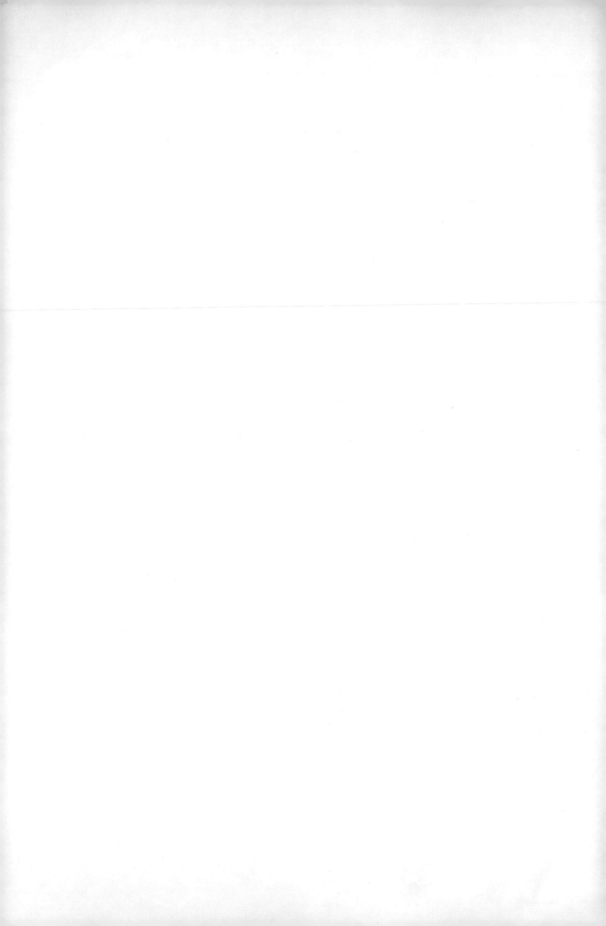